CHINESE
MEDICINE
CURES

HEADACHES

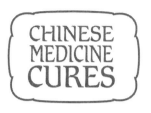

HEADACHES

BOB FLAWS

Adapted for the UK by Sylvia Schroer

foulsham

LONDON • NEW YORK • TORONTO • SYDNEY

foulsham

The Publishing House, Bennetts Close,
Cippenham, Berkshire SL1 5AP, England

ISBN 0-572-02590-4

Copyright © 1998 and 1999 Blue Poppy Press, USA
This UK revised edition copyright © 2000 W. Foulsham and Co. Ltd

Cover photograph © The Image Bank

Printed in Great Britain by St. Edmundsbury Press, Bury St. Edmunds, Suffolk

CONTENTS

PREFACE

This book is a layperson's introduction to Chinese medicine and headaches. It covers the Chinese theories about what causes headaches as well as the diagnosis and treatment of headaches with acupuncture and Chinese herbal medicine. In addition, it includes a host of inexpensive or free home remedies and suggestions as to how to prevent and treat headaches. These remedies include Chinese dietary therapy, Chinese self-massage, Chinese herbal teas, wines and porridges, moxibustion, aromatherapy, herbal inhalants, hydrotherapy and poultices and plasters.

Based on my 20 years of clinical experience and as an occasional migraine sufferer myself, I believe that Chinese medicine is extremely effective for curing – not just relieving – the majority of chronic, recurrent headaches. Not only can it relieve the localised pain and pressure but, because it treats by returning the entire person to a more harmonious state of balance, people generally report that they feel healthier and better in themselves.

Chinese medicine is a rising star in the realm of alternative or complementary therapy in the world today, and rightly so. As the oldest, continually practised, literate, professional medicine in the world, Chinese medicine is a vast treasure house filled with wise theories and compassionate treatments. I have written this book in the hope that more Westerners will try Chinese medicine and see what it can do for them.

Bob Flaws

INTRODUCTION

ean has hidden herself in her bedroom, door closed, lights off, and the curtains tightly shut. The left side of her head is pounding, she feels sick, and she cannot stand any noise or light. Two hours earlier, she felt a familiar numb sensation on the side of her mouth, followed by tingling in her hands and a narrowing of her field of vision. When she felt these sensations, she knew she was in for another one of her 'killer' migraines. For several hours she will be in agony. Eventually, she will vomit and have diarrhoea. After that, she will fall asleep. When she wakes up tomorrow, she will feel as if she has been through a wringer, but at least she can go back to work. This same scenario plays itself out several times per year. Over-the-counter Western headache medicine doesn't touch Jean's pain, and she is afraid to use stronger Western prescription drugs.

In the case above, Jean is having a pretty severe migraine headache. Your headaches may not be so severe. Perhaps yours is more of a tension headache. However, whatever the type of headache you suffer from, Chinese medicine can probably help you either to eliminate the headaches altogether or, at the least, to minimise their frequency and severity. Chinese medicine has records going back over 2,000 years dealing with the treatment of all kinds of headaches. During that time, 100 generations of highly skilled and trained practitioners have written down their experiences in treating headaches with acupuncture, Chinese herbal medicine and a number of other Asian treatment methods. There have also been many research studies conducted since 1949 in the People's Republic of China on the Chinese medical treatment of this all-too-common complaint. It is a well established fact that Chinese medicine does treat headaches very effectively.

SOME INFORMATION ON WESTERN MEDICINE AND HEADACHES

Before we look into the Chinese medical description of the causes and treatment of headaches, it is useful first to introduce a little basic information on what Western medicine has to say about headaches, particularly since this book has been written mainly for people living in the Western world.

The two most common types of headache according to Western research are tension headaches and migraines. Tension headaches are typified by a dull, steady, non-throbbing pain, usually felt on the front of the head or on both sides. This pain may be either mild or severe. Sometimes, your head may feel as though it is in the grip of a vice or is being squeezed by a tight band. Sometimes, the pain extends to the neck and shoulders. Such tension headaches may last one to two hours or all day. They often occur in the late afternoon or evening as a result of stress accumulated during the day. Some people may have chronic tension headaches that occur on a daily or almost daily basis and this may go on for months and even years. According to Western medicine, the cause of this kind of tension headache is emotional stress resulting in tightening of the muscles of the head and neck. However, tension headaches may also be caused by poor posture, remaining in the same position for too long, or arthritis.

Migraine headaches, on the other hand, are characterised by moderate to severe pounding or throbbing pain, most commonly felt on only one side of the head. Often, these one-sided headaches are accompanied by nausea, vomiting, dizziness and hypersensitivity to light and/or sound. About 10–15 per cent of migraine sufferers experience an 'aura' or 'prodrome' before the pain in their heads begins. These auras include visual disturbances, such as flashing spots, colours, lines or shapes, or temporary reductions in their field of vision, such as tunnel vision. When head pain is preceded by such distortions in vision, this is called a classic migraine, while so-called common migraines are not preceded by any visual auras. Although as many as 25 per cent of the population probably experience a migraine at least once in their life, 70 per cent of migraine sufferers are women. Migraines may last from a few hours to three days and may come only a couple of times in a lifetime or several times a week. The average number of attacks is one to three times per month and attacks often correspond to certain times in the menstrual cycle in women. Nine out of ten migraine sufferers have a close relative who suffers from migraines.

In those who are predisposed to get them, migraines may be triggered by certain foods, alcohol and caffeine. Changes in weather or sleep patterns, skipped meals, some medications and stress all play a part to varying degrees in different individuals and bright lights, cigarette smoke, intense heat and loud noises can also precipitate an attack in some people. Further, there is a link between migraines and oral birth-control pills and hormone replacement therapy in menopausal women.

Apart from these two main types of headaches, there are several others worth mentioning. Cluster headaches are relatively uncommon but, when they occur, they can cause excruciating, knife-like pain around or in one eye. They are called cluster headaches because sufferers typically will have an attack every day, usually at the same time, for several weeks or months. Then they disappear for months or even years. Nine out of ten cluster headache patients are men.

Rebound headaches occur in patients who have overused headache medications to relieve persistent headache pain. In this case, the medication that was taken to get rid of the pain actually starts to make the headache worse.

Another cause of pain in the head and face is sinusitis. The sufferer typically has a green, pussy, nasal discharge, nasal congestion and tenderness over the affected sinus. Often the pain is worse in the morning and aggravated by cold, damp weather. There is commonly a recent history of cold or hay fever.

Very occasionally, headaches can indicate a more severe health problem or illness that should be investigated.

EAST IS EAST AND WEST IS WEST

Chinese medicine is a system of medical thought and practice distinct and separate from modern Western medicine. This means that one must shift one's models of reality when it comes to thinking about Chinese medicine. It has taken the Chinese more than 2,000 years to develop this medical system. Having spent the last 20 years of my life both practising and writing and teaching about Chinese medicine in the West, I feel very strongly that Chinese medicine is best understood on its own terms rather than by trying to explain it according to Western medical science.

Most people reading this book probably have some basic knowledge of biology. Whether we recognise it or not, most of us Westerners think of what we learned about the human body at school as the one true description of reality, not just one possible interpretation. If Chinese medicine is to make any sense to Westerners at all, we need to accept the notion that there are other valid descriptions of the human body and its functions, and of health and disease. In grappling with this fundamentally important issue, it is useful to think about the concepts of a map and the terrain it describes.

If we take the United Kingdom as an example, we can have numerous different maps of this country's land mass. One map might show population. Another might show per capita incomes. Another might simply be a road map. We could also show political or county boundaries. In fact, there could be an infinite number of potentially different maps of the United Kingdom, depending on what you were trying to show and do. As long as the map is based on accurate information and has been created with self-consistent logic, then one map is not necessarily more correct than another. The issue is to use the right map for what you are trying to do. If you wanted to drive from London to Glasgow, for example, a road map is probably the best one for the job, but is not necessarily a truer or more real description of the United Kingdom than a map showing annual rainfall.

The point I am trying to make is that the map is not the terrain. The Western biological map of the human body is only one potentially useful medical map. It is no more true than the traditional Chinese medical map, and the facts of one map cannot be reduced to the criteria or standards of another unless they share the same logic right from the beginning. As long as the Western medical map is capable of solving a person's disease in a cost-effective, time-efficient manner without side-effects or iatrogenesis (disease or illness caused by a treatment), then it is a useful map. Chinese medicine needs to be judged in the same way. The Chinese medical map of health and disease is just as real and every bit as useful as the Western biological map as long as, in using it, practitioners and patients are able to solve health problems in a safe and effective way.

The following chapter is an introduction to the basics of Chinese medicine. Unless you understand some of the fundamental theories and principles of Chinese medicine, you will not be able to understand or accept the reasons for some of the Chinese medical treatments of headaches.

AN OVERVIEW OF THE CHINESE MEDICAL MAP

In this chapter, we will look at an overview of Chinese medicine. In particular, we will discuss yin and yang, qi and blood, essence and spirit, the viscera and bowels, and the channels and network vessels. In the following chapter, we will look at the concept of pain in Chinese medicine. Once we understand these things, we can then go on to see how Chinese medicine views headaches and how practitioners of Chinese medicine diagnose and treat various patterns of headache. Should you find any of the language or terms used difficult to understand, there is a glossary on pages 159–64 to which you can refer.

YIN AND YANG

To understand Chinese medicine, one must first understand the concepts of yin and yang since these are the most basic concepts in this system. Yin and yang are the cornerstones for understanding, diagnosing and treating the body and mind in Chinese medicine. In a sense, all the other theories and concepts of Chinese medicine are nothing other than an elaboration of yin and yang. Most people have probably already heard of yin and yang but may not have a clear idea of what these terms mean.

The concepts of yin and yang can be used to describe everything that exists in the universe, including all the parts and functions of the body. Originally, yin referred to the shady side of a hill and yang to the sunny side of the hill. Since sunshine and shade are two interdependent sides of a single reality, these two aspects of the hill are seen as part of a single whole. Other examples of yin and yang are that night exists only in relation to day and cold exists only in relation to heat. According to Chinese thought, every single thing that exists in the universe has these two aspects, a yin and a yang. Thus everything has a front and a back, a top and a bottom, a left and a right, and a beginning and an end. However, something is yin or yang only in relation to its paired complement. Nothing is of itself yin or yang.

It is the concepts of yin and yang that make Chinese medicine a holistic medicine. This is because, based on this unitary and complementary vision of reality, no body part or body function is viewed as separate or isolated from the whole person. The table below shows a partial list of yin and yang pairs as they apply to the body. It is vital to remember that each item listed is either yin or yang only in relation to its complementary partner. Nothing is absolutely or within itself either yin or yang. As we can see, it is possible to describe every aspect of the body in terms of yin and yang.

Yin	Yang
Form	Function
Organs	Bowels
Blood	Qi
Inside	Outside
Front of body	Back of body
Right side	Left side
Lower body	Upper body
Cool, cold	Warm, hot
Stillness	Activity, movement

QI AND BLOOD

Qi (pronounced chee) and blood make up the most important complementary pair of yin and yang within the human body. It is said that, in the world, yin and yang are water and fire but, in the human body, yin and yang are blood and qi. Qi is yang in relation to blood, which is yin.

Qi

Qi is often translated as energy and certainly energy is a manifestation of qi. Chinese language scholars would say, however, that qi is larger than any single type of energy described by modern Western science. Paul Unschuld, perhaps one of the greatest living sinologists, translates the word qi as influences. This conveys the sense that qi is responsible for change and movement. So with regard to Chinese medicine, qi is that which motivates all movement and transformation or change.

In Chinese medicine, qi is defined as having five specific functions:

1. Defence
It is qi that is responsible for protecting the exterior of the body from invasion by external pathogens. This qi, called defensive qi, flows through the outer part of the body.

2. Transformation
Qi transforms substances so that they can be utilised by the body. An example of this function is the transformation of the food we eat into nutrients to nourish the body, which then produces more qi and blood.

3. Warmth
Qi, being relatively yang, is inherently warm, and one of the main functions of the qi is to warm the entire body, both

inside and out. If this warming function of the qi is weak, cold may cause the flow of qi and blood to be congealed in a similar way to the effect of cold on water – freezing.

4. Restraint
It is qi that holds all the organs and substances in their proper places. Thus all the organs, blood and fluids need qi to keep them from falling or leaking out of their specific pathways. If this function of the qi is weak, then problems like uterine prolapse, a tendency to bruise easily or urinary incontinence may occur.

5. Transportation
Qi provides the motivating force for all transportation and movement in the body. Every aspect of the body that moves is moved by the qi. The qi moves the blood and body fluids throughout the body. It moves food through the stomach and blood through the vessels.

Blood
In Chinese medicine, blood refers to the red fluid that flows through our vessels as in modern Western medicine, but it also has different meanings and implications. Most basically, blood is the substance that nourishes and moistens all the body tissues. Without blood, body tissues cannot function properly. Additionally, when there is insufficient blood or it is scanty, body tissues become dry and wither.

Qi and blood are closely interrelated. It is said, 'Qi is the commander of the blood and blood is the mother of qi.' This means that it is qi that moves the blood but that it is the blood that provides the nourishment and physical foundation for the creation and existence of the qi.

In Chinese medicine, blood provides the following functions for the body:

1. Nourishment

Blood nourishes the body. Along with qi, the blood goes to every part of the body. When the blood is deficient, function decreases and tissues atrophy or shrink.

2. Moistening

Blood moistens the body tissues. This includes the skin, eyes, and ligaments and tendons or what are in Chinese medicine simply called the sinews of body. A deficiency or lack of blood can cause drying-out and consequent stiffening of various body tissues throughout the body.

3. Blood provides the material foundation for the spirit or mind

In Chinese medicine, the body and mind are considered as one. The spirit is considered to be a great accumulation of qi. The blood (yin) supplies the material support and nourishment for the spirit (yang) so that it accumulates, becomes bright (i.e. conscious and clever), and stays rooted in the body. If the blood becomes deficient, the mind can 'float', causing problems like insomnia, agitation and unrest.

ESSENCE

Along with qi and blood, essence is one of the three most important constituents of the body. Essence is the most fundamental, essential material the body uses for its growth, maturation and reproduction. There are two forms of this essence. We inherit essence from our parents and we also produce our own essence from the food and drink we consume and the air we breathe.

The essence that comes from our parents is what determines our basic constitution, strength and vitality. We each have a finite, limited amount of this inherited essence. It is important to protect and conserve this essence because all bodily functions depend upon it and, when it is gone, we die. The depletion of essence has serious implications for our overall health and well-being. Fortunately, the essence derived from food and drink helps to bolster and support this inherited essence. So, if we eat well and do not consume more qi and blood than we create each day, then when we sleep at night this surplus qi and, more especially, blood is transformed into essence.

It is said in Chinese medicine that essence is stored 'in the kidneys'. The actual location where the kidneys store this essence is not necessarily in the kidneys themselves but may also be in other tissues associated with the kidneys. For example, it is said that stored essence becomes the marrow. Marrow in Chinese medicine means the bone marrow but also the nerves found in the spine, while the brain itself is called the sea of marrow. We will see below that essence plays an important role in at least one kind of headache based on the principle that the brain is the sea of marrow.

SPIRIT

Spirit in Chinese medicine means one's mental–emotional faculties. Basically, it is a way of saying consciousness. In Chinese medicine, this term does not have any religious or 'spiritual' connotation. Spirit in a Chinese medical sense is seen as an accumulation of qi and blood in the heart. If sufficient qi and blood accumulate in the heart, then this gives rise to consciousness, which, according to Chinese medicine, is called the spirit. Due to the close relationship between the essence, the qi and the spirit, sometimes consciousness is called the essence spirit. If we are talking particularly about the emotions, then the compound term 'spirit will' ('will' here means 'desire') is commonly used. At other times, because the spirit is associated with mental clarity, the compound term 'spirit brightness' or 'spirit brilliance' is used. In order for there to be spirit, there must be sufficient qi. In order for the spirit to be calm and healthy, there must be sufficient blood to nourish the spirit and keep it under control. Since the spirit made from qi is inherently yang in nature, it tends to stir or become restless if yin blood does not nourish and 'mother' it. So, normal mental clarity is referred to as 'having spirit', while emotional turmoil is referred to as 'spirit not quiet' or 'restless spirit'.

On the one hand, the spirit is made up from the qi and blood that are produced by the viscera and bowels we will talk about next. On the other, the qi and, therefore, the spirit are affected by external stimuli. Thus, there is no dichotomy or division in Chinese medicine between the psychological and biological. The mind arises as a function of the viscera and bowels, but the functioning of the viscera and bowels is affected by the experiences of the mind and emotions. In fact, every thought in the mind or felt emotion relates to a corresponding movement of qi. If we change the way the qi moves, we change our mental and emotional experience, whilst changing our mind and emotions changes the way the qi moves. Thus the qi and the spirit or mind are not seen as two different things but rather a single reality.

THE VISCERA AND BOWELS

In Chinese medicine, the internal organs (called viscera so as not to become confused with the Western biological entities of the same name) have a wider area of function and influence than in Western medicine. Each viscus has distinct responsibilities for maintaining the physical and psychological health of the individual. When thinking about the internal viscera according to Chinese medicine, it is more accurate to view them as spheres of influence or a network that spreads throughout the body, rather than as a distinct and separate physical organ as described by Western science. This is why the famous German sinologist, Manfred Porkert, refers to them as orbs rather than organs. In Chinese medicine, the relationship between the various viscera and other parts of the body is made possible by the channel and network vessel system that we will discuss later.

In Chinese medicine, there are five main viscera that are relatively yin, and six main bowels that are relatively yang. The five yin viscera are the heart, lungs, liver, spleen and kidneys. The six yang bowels are the stomach, small intestine, large intestine, gall bladder, urinary bladder and a system that Chinese medicine refers to as the triple burner. All the functions of the entire body are categorised or described under these eleven organs or spheres of influence. Chinese medicine as a system does not have a pancreas, a pituitary gland, or ovaries. All the functions of these Western organs are contained in the Chinese medical system of the five viscera and six bowels.

Visceral correspondences

Within this system, the five viscera are the most important. These are the organs that Chinese medicine says are responsible for the creation and transformation of qi and blood and the storage of essence. For example, the kidneys are responsible for the excretion of urine but are also responsible for hearing, the strength of the bones, sex, reproduction, maturation and growth, the lower and upper back, the lower legs in general and particularly the knees. This demonstrates that the Chinese viscera may have the same name and even some overlapping functions but still are quite different from the organs of modern Western medicine. Each of the five Chinese medical viscera also has a corresponding tissue, sense and emotion related to it. These are outlined in the table below.

Organ	Tissue	Sense	Spirit	Emotion
Lungs	Skin/body hair	Smell	Corporeal soul	Grief/sadness
Spleen	Flesh	Taste	Thought	Thinking/worry
Kidneys	Bones/head hair	Hearing	Will	Fear
Liver	Sinews	Sight	Ethereal soul	Anger
Heart	Blood vessels	Speech	Spirit	Joy/fright

In addition, each Chinese medical viscus or bowel possesses both a yin and a yang aspect. The yin aspect of a viscus or bowel refers to its substantial nature or tangible form. Further, an organ's yin is responsible for the nurturing, cooling and moistening of that viscus or bowel. The yang aspect of the viscus or bowel represents its functional activities or what it does. An organ's yang aspect is also warming. These two aspects, yin and yang, form and function, cooling and heating, create good health when balanced. If either yin or yang becomes too strong or too weak, the resulting imbalance may lead to disease.

Four out of five of the viscera may be associated with the causes and mechanisms of headaches. These are the liver, spleen, heart and kidneys. Only two of the six bowels are associated with headaches in Chinese medicine, the gall bladder and the stomach. Described over the next pages are the main principles of Chinese medicine regarding these four viscera and two bowels that we will be using in our study of the diagnosis and treatment of headaches.

The kidneys

In Chinese medicine, the kidneys are considered to be the foundation of our life. Since the developing foetus is shaped like a kidney and as the kidneys are the main viscus for the storage of inherited essence, the kidneys are referred to as the prenatal root. Keeping the kidney qi strong and kidney yin and yang in relative balance is considered essential to good health and longevity. According to Chinese medicine the aspects of kidneys that are relevant to the mechanisms of headache are:

1. Human reproduction, development and maturation

These are the same functions we used when describing the essence. This is because the essence is stored in the kidneys. Health problems related to reproduction, development and maturation are considered to be problems of the kidney essence. Excessive sexual activity, drug use and simple prolonged exhaustion can all damage and consume kidney essence. Kidney essence is also consumed by the process of ageing.

2. Water metabolism

The kidneys work in co-ordination with the lungs and spleen to ensure that water is spread properly throughout the body and that excess water is excreted as urination. Problems such as oedema (swelling due to water retention), excessive dryness or excessive urination can indicate a weakness of kidney function.

3. Storing the will

Will in this sense is best translated as desire. If kidney qi is insufficient, this aspect of our human nature can be weakened. Conversely, pushing ourselves to extremes, for example by long-distance running or cycling, can eventually exhaust our kidneys.

4. Fear
Fear can manifest when the kidney qi is insufficient. On the other hand, constant or excessive fear can damage the kidneys and make them weak.

5. Bones, marrow and brain
According to Chinese medicine, the kidneys govern the bones, the bones engender the marrow, and the brain is the sea of marrow. This means that there is a very close relationship between kidney essence and the brain. If kidney essence becomes insufficient, the brain may lose its nourishment.

6. The lower back
Chinese medicine calls the lower back the 'mansion of the kidneys', mansion meaning the realm of influence. If the kidneys become weak and vacuous, then lower back pain is one of the key symptoms of this imbalance.

7. The liver
The kidneys are said to be the 'mother' of the liver. In particular, it is kidney yin or kidney water that moistens and enriches the liver, keeping the liver soft and harmonious.

The liver
In Chinese medicine, the liver is associated with our emotional state, some aspects of digestion and with menstruation in women. Specifically, aspects of its functions include:

1. Coursing and discharge
Coursing and discharge refer to the uninhibited spreading of qi to every part of the body. If the liver is not able to maintain the free and smooth flow of qi throughout the body, multiple physical and emotional symptoms can develop. This function

of the liver is most easily damaged by emotional causes and, in particular, by inappropriate anger and frustration. For example, if the liver is stressed due to pent-up anger, the flow of liver qi can become depressed or stagnate.

Liver qi stagnation can cause a wide range of health problems, including PMS (premenstrual stress), chronic digestive disturbance, depression and insomnia. So, it is essential to keep our liver qi flowing freely.

2. Storing the blood
The liver regulates the amount of blood in circulation. When the body is at rest, the blood in the extremities returns to the liver. It is said in Chinese medicine that the liver is yin in form but yang in function. This means that the liver requires sufficient blood to keep it and its associated tissues moist and supple, cool and relaxed, i.e. yin in form.

3. Anger
Inappropriate anger is the emotion that typically arises when the liver is diseased and when its qi does not flow freely. Anger, like all our emotions, is essential to our health and well-being. Learning how to listen to anger within ourselves and in turn use its powerful energy to transform our lives is a lifelong challenge. Having a healthy liver is really important in this regard. If anger is not dealt with, it can turn into rage, frustration and depression. If there is stagnation of qi in the liver, then it will be all the more likely that we experience these negative forms of anger. Conversely, anger and frustration can damage the liver.

4. Upbearing and effusion
As long as the liver courses and discharges the qi, the qi moves upwards and outwards in a healthy and harmonious way. If the liver qi becomes depressed and stagnant, it may

eventually vent itself upwards (due to its yang nature) in a pathological way. Most pathological upward counterflow of qi is associated in Chinese medicine with the liver. As we will see later, pathological upward counterflow of qi to the head is a main cause of headaches.

The heart

The heart's role in the cause and mechanisms of headaches primarily revolves around its role in the creation and control of blood. The basic functons of the heart in Chinese medicine that relate to the blood are:

1. Governing the blood

It is the heart qi that 'stirs' or moves the blood within its vessels. This is roughly analogous to the idea that the heart is a pump for the blood in Western medicine. The pulsation of the blood through the arteries due to the contraction of the heart is referred to as the 'stirring of the pulse'. The Chinese word for 'pulse' and 'vessel' is the same, so this could also be translated as the 'stirring of the vessels'.

2. Storing the spirit

The spirit in this sense means the mind. The heart is said to be the place where the spirit is stored, so mental function, mental clarity and mental equilibrium are all associated with the heart. If the heart does not receive enough qi or blood or if the heart is disturbed by something, the spirit may become restless and this may produce symptoms of mental or emotional unrest, heart palpitations and insomnia. Frequent, vivid dreams are another symptom of a restless spirit.

3. Governing the vessels

This is very similar to point 1 above. The vessels here refer to the blood vessels and also to the pulse.

The spleen

Since at least the Yuan dynasty (1280–1368 AD), the spleen has been considered to be one of the two most important viscera of Chinese medicine (the other being the kidneys). In Chinese medicine, the spleen plays a pivotal role in the creation of qi and blood and in the circulation and transformation of body fluids. The role of the spleen in Chinese medicine is very wide-reaching and more important than in Western medicine. This is an excellent illustration of how these two systems of medicine differ in their views of the internal organs and their functions. The main functions of the spleen according to Chinese medicine that relate to headaches are:

1. Governing movement and transformation
This refers firstly to the movement and transformation of foods and liquids through the digestive system and really means digestion. It also refers to the movement and transformation of body fluids through the body. The spleen qi is largely responsible for controlling liquid metabolism in the body.

2. Restraining the blood
As mentioned earlier, one of the five functions of the qi is to restrain the fluids of the body, including the blood, within their proper channels and reservoirs. If the spleen qi is healthy and abundant, then the blood is held within its vessels properly. Should the spleen qi become weak and deficient, then the blood may flow outside its channels and vessels resulting in various types of pathological bleeding. This includes bleeding associated with the menstrual cycle.

3. Storing the constructive
The 'constructive' here refers to a type of qi in the body. Specifically, it is the qi responsible for nourishing and

constructing the body and its tissues. This constructive qi is closely associated with the process of digestion and the creation of qi and blood out of food and liquids. If the spleen fails to store or runs out of constructive qi, then the person becomes hungry and, eventually, fatigued.

4. Thought

In the West, we do not usually think of the process of thought as an emotion as such. It is difficult to find an exact translation for this term: perhaps 'worry' or 'over-thinking' give a better idea of what it means. Excessive thinking and worry cause the spleen qi to bind. This means that the spleen qi does not flow harmoniously and this typically manifests in symptoms such as loss of appetite, abdominal bloating after meals and indigestion.

5. Engenderment and transformation

Engenderment and transformation refer to the creation or production of the qi and blood out of the food and drink we take in each day. If the spleen receives adequate food and drink and transforms them properly, it engenders or creates the qi and blood. The kidneys and lungs also participate in the creation of the qi, whilst the kidneys and heart participate in the creation of the blood. However, the spleen is the pivotal viscus in both processes, and spleen qi weakness and insufficiency is a major cause of qi and blood insufficiency and weakness.

The gall bladder

The main functions of the gall bladder in terms of headaches in Chinese medicine are:

1. Governing decision

In Chinese medicine, the liver is likened to a general who plans strategy for the body, while the gall bladder is likened to a judge. According to this point of view, if a person lacks gall bladder qi, they will have trouble making decisions. Additionally, they will have a timid or hesitant demeanour. While courage in the West is often associated with the heart (the word for courage is derived from *coeur*, the French for heart), bravery in the East is frequently associated with the gall bladder. Actually, this is also an old Western idea as well. When someone is very forward and brazen, we say that they have gall. According to Chinese medicine if someone is excessively timid, this may be due to gall bladder qi vacuity or insufficiency.

2. Forming a yin–yang pair with the liver

This underlines the particularly close relationship between the liver and the gall bladder. If the liver becomes diseased, this often manifests along the pathways of the gall bladder channel.

The stomach

The stomach is important in Chinese medicine due to its pivotal role in digestion and, therefore, in the creation of qi and blood. Here we will only outline the functions relevant to our discussion of the disease causes and disease mechanisms of headache in Chinese medicine.

1. Governing intake

This means that the stomach is the first to receive foods and drinks ingested into the body.

2. Downbearing of the turbid

The process of digestion in Chinese medicine is likened to the process of fermentation and then distillation. The stomach is the fermentation tun in which food and liquids rot and ripen. This rotting and ripening allows for the separation of 'clear' and 'turbid' parts of the digested substances. The spleen sends the clear parts upward to the lungs and heart to become the qi and blood respectively. The stomach sends the turbid part down to be excreted from the large intestine and bladder.

3. Harmony and downbearing

The normal movement of the stomach's qi is downwards. If the stomach becomes diseased, its qi frequently counterflows upwards. This results in nausea and vomiting. If liver qi counterflows upwards, this can easily carry the stomach qi upwards along with it. An extension of this is the statement that 'The stomach is the central pivot for the upbearing and downbearing of yin and yang.' Any disease affecting the stomach may affect normal upbearing and downbearing, while any disease of the stomach may affect the upbearing and downbearing of the rest of the body.

The triple burner

It is said in Chinese medicine: 'The triple burner has a function but no form.' The name refers to the three main areas of the torso. The upper burner is the chest. The middle burner is the space from the bottom of the rib-cage to the level of the navel. The lower burner is the lower abdomen below the navel. These three spaces are called burners because all of the functions and transformations of the viscera and bowels that they contain are 'warm' transformations. This transformation process is thought to be like food cooking in a pot on a stove or an alchemical transformation in a furnace. The triple burner is really a general concept of how the other viscera and bowels function together as an organic unit in terms of the digestion of foods and liquids and the circulation and transformation of body fluids.

The channels and network vessels

Each viscus and bowel has a corresponding channel or meridian with which it is connected. In Chinese medicine, the inside of the body is made up of the viscera and bowels. The outside of the body is composed of the sinews and bones, muscles, flesh, skin and hair. It is the channels and network vessels (i.e. smaller, connecting vessels) that connect the inside and the outside of the body. It is through these channels and network vessels that the viscera and bowels connect with their corresponding body tissues.

The channels and network vessel system is a unique feature of traditional Chinese medicine. These channels and vessels are different from the circulatory, nervous or lymphatic systems. The earliest reference to these channels and vessels is in *Nei Jing (The Inner Classic)*, a text written around the second or third century BC.

The channels and vessels perform two basic functions. They are the pathways by which the qi and blood circulate through the body and between the organs and tissues. Additionally, as mentioned above, the channels connect the viscera and bowels internally with the exterior part of the body. This channel and vessel system functions in the body much like an information or communication network. The channels allow the various parts of our body to co-operate and interact to maintain our lives.

This channel and network vessel system is quite complex. There are 12 primary channels, six yin and six yang, each with a specific pathway through the external body and connected with an internal organ (see diagram opposite). There are also extraordinary vessels, sinew channels, channel divergences, main network vessels and ultimately countless finer and finer network vessels permeating the entire body. All of these form a closed loop or circuit similar to but distinct from the Western circulatory system.

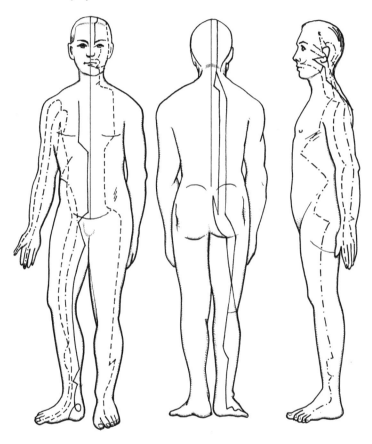

Acupuncture points are places located on the major channels where there is a special concentration of qi and blood. Because of the relatively greater quantity of qi and blood accumulated at these places, the sites act as switches that can potentially control the flow of qi and blood in the channel on which the point is located. By stimulating these points in different ways, one can speed up or slow down, make more or reduce, warm or cool the qi and blood flowing in the channels and vessels. The main ways of stimulating these points and thus adjusting the flow of qi and blood in the channels and vessels is to manipulate them with needles (see page 81) or heat them by moxibustion (see page 117). Other commonly used ways of stimulating these points and thus adjusting the qi and blood flowing through the channels and vessels are massage, cupping, the application of magnets and the application of various herbal medicinals. If the channels and vessels are the pathways over which the qi and blood flow, then the acupuncture points are the places where this flow can be adjusted.

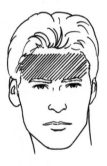
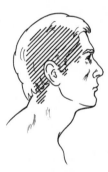

Yang ming area   *Shao yang area*

The area of the head is divided into four general regions in terms of Chinese channels. The forehead and front of the face are the areas traversed by the *yang ming* channels. The *yang ming* refers to the large intestine and stomach channels. The sides of the head are traversed by the *shao yang* channels. The *shao yang* refers to the gall bladder and triple burner channels. The back of the head is the area traversed by the *tai yang*. The *tai yang* refers to the bladder and small intestine channels, both of which connect with the governing vessel, which is usually also involved in headaches affecting this part of the head. The top of the head is where an internal branch of the *jue yin* ends. In terms of headache the *jue yin* means the liver channel.

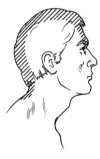

Tai yang area

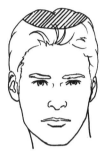

Jue yin area

PAIN IN CHINESE MEDICINE

here is a basic dictum in Chinese medicine about pain, which covers all types of pain felt anywhere in the body for any reason. The saying goes, 'If there is pain, there is no free flow; if there is free flow, there is no pain.' In other words, pain is the body's immediate sensation of a lack of free flow of the qi, blood and body fluids. As long as the qi, blood and body fluids are freely and smoothly flowing, there is no experience of pain.

Two conditions may cause a lack of free flow: either something is blocking and obstructing free flow or there is not enough qi or blood to flow freely. This means that these two factors are the only two fundamental causes of any pain felt anywhere in the body. It does not matter whether the pain is strong or weak, instantaneous or lingering, sharp or dull, localised or wide-ranging; in Chinese medicine there are only these two reasons for pain.

BLOCKAGE AND OBSTRUCTION

The first main cause of lack of free flow and, therefore, of pain is blockage and obstruction. This means that there is sufficient qi and blood to flow freely, but something has become stagnant and gathered. Thus the qi and blood flow is hindered and blocked.

Internal causes

There are six things that may become blocked and inhibit free flow in the body, referred to as the six depressions. They are qi, blood, dampness, phlegm, food and fire.

As we have seen, if the liver loses its control over coursing and discharging, the qi will not spread freely throughout the body. It stagnates and accumulates. This is mainly due to what in Chinese is referred to as 'the emotions not being fulfilled'. The implication of this is that all our emotions, which are seen as the subjective feelings associated with various desires, put the qi in motion. If the desire is fulfilled, the qi can run its course. If the desire cannot be fulfilled, the movement of qi towards or away from the object of its desire is thwarted. This thwarting of our desires or emotions causes the liver to lose its function and the qi to become stagnant and depressed. The qi fails to flow freely, and this can cause pain.

In Chinese medicine it is said, 'The qi moves the blood. If the qi moves, the blood moves. If the qi stops, the blood stops.' If there is liver depression qi stagnation due to emotional stress and frustration, then, over time, this will also lead to blood stasis. Static blood is also a lack of free flow. So static blood, or blood stasis, is another cause of pain. Static blood may also be directly caused by traumatic injury. If static blood due to traumatic injury is not dispersed it will impede the flow of qi, since the qi and blood flow together. In this case, static blood, which is yin and substantial, impedes the free flow of yang qi, which is insubstantial and cannot penetrate the accumulated static blood.

Just as qi and blood flow together and form a yin–yang pair, body fluids also flow through the body and have a reciprocal relationship with both the qi and blood. The qi moves and transforms body fluids. If the qi becomes stagnant, then body fluids may also accumulate, just as the blood becomes static. If body fluids accumulate pathologically and are not moved and transformed, these are referred to as damp depression. Conversely, if for any reason, dampness is formed, it may hinder and obstruct the free flow of qi and blood. The qi cannot move through this yin dampness and it is said that blood and body fluids flow together. If one stops, so will the other. As damp depression may cause lack of free flow, dampness can also be a cause of pain.

If dampness gathers and lingers for a long time, or if it is transformed by either heat or cold, it may turn into phlegm. Phlegm is simply congealed dampness. No matter what the cause of phlegm, once it is produced, it may hinder the free flow of the qi and blood. So it too may be associated with pain due to obstruction and impediment of free flow.

Qi is supposed to move and transform not only blood and body fluids but also food. If the qi becomes depressed and stagnant, the digestate may not be moved. This yin substance then further blocks the free flow of qi and blood, and causes pain. This pain mostly occurs in the stomach and abdomen, so it is not a main cause of headache. However, if food becomes stagnant and accumulates for any reason, then this can aggravate any other cause or tendency to qi, blood, damp or phlegm obstruction.

Qi is yang in nature and is therefore warm. If qi becomes depressed and accumulates, a lot of yang qi in one place may give rise to pathological heat. If there is enough heat, this is called evil fire. The nature of fire is to flare or flame upwards. So depressive heat produced in the internal viscera, such as the liver, gall bladder and stomach, often moves upwards to accumulate in the head. If it becomes blocked there in the 'bony box' of the skull, it will prevent the healthy or so-called righteous qi and blood from moving freely. There will be pain.

External causes
It is also possible for obstruction and blockage to be caused by what Chinese medicine calls external evils. If external pathogens (evils) invade the body, they lodge in places where they are not meant to be. It is a basic axiom that two things cannot inhabit the same space: if one exists there, the other cannot. In the same way, external evils that invade the body block and hinder the free flow of the righteous qi and blood. This results in pain.

Different natures, different types of pain

Depending on what is obstructed and what is doing the obstructing, there are different types of pain. For example, qi stagnation causes distended, bloated feelings of discomfort. Static blood is associated with fixed, localised pain, which is sharp or piercing in nature or simply very severe in intensity. Dampness causes heavy, distended, tight pain. Phlegm itself typically is painless. However, because it can block the free flow of qi and blood, phlegm obstruction may be associated with pain of either type. Pain associated with externally invading wind evils moves about, comes and goes, and mostly affects the upper body. It may also be associated with tingling, itching or numbness. Pain associated with cold is typically fixed in location, intense and chilly in nature. It is improved by warmth. Pain associated with heat or fire is hot in nature and can also be quite intense. Apart from heat, pain, and redness, there may also be swelling.

Pain that is due to something blocking and obstructing the free flow of qi and blood is called replete pain in Chinese medicine.

INSUFFICIENCY AND WEAKNESS

The lack of free flow may also be because of either a lack of qi to move blood and body fluids or a lack of blood to fill the vessels. If qi vacuity and weakness is even more severe, it is called yang vacuity. Yang is merely a lot of qi in one place. If blood vacuity is more severe, it is called yin and/or essence insufficiency. Yin is nothing other than a lot of blood and essence in one place. Lack of free flow due to vacuity and insufficiency is called vacuity pain. Vacuity pain is typically not as severe as replete pain. However, it tends to be enduring and persistent and is aggravated by exertion, fatigue and loss of blood or body fluids.

Mixed repletion and vacuity

In real life, the body is very complex, and most people with disease present a mixture of vacuity and repletion. For example, if the spleen qi becomes vacuous and weak, the qi may not move and transform body fluids. These then give rise to phlegm and dampness, which obstruct and hinder the free flow of qi and blood. It is also possible for blood vacuity to give rise to blood stasis or blood stasis to give rise to blood vacuity. If there is insufficient blood to nourish and construct the vessels, the vessels may not perform their job of moving the blood. This leads to the creation of static blood. In addition, another term for static blood is dry or dead blood. Static blood inhibits the engenderment and transformation of new or fresh blood. If blood vacuity persists for long enough, it will give rise to yin vacuity, since blood is part of yin fluids and essence. This illustrates why our pain can be a mixture of both vacuity and repletion causes and mechanisms.

How to stop pain using Chinese medicine

If all pain in the body can be reduced to lack of free flow, then all pain in the body can be treated by restoring the free flow. 'If there is pain, there is no free flow. If there is free flow, there is no pain.' So the basic principle in Chinese medicine for stopping or alleviating pain is to promote the free flow. In order to achieve this we need to know whether that pain is due to obstruction and blockage or due to weakness and insufficiency. If it is due to obstruction and blockage, then we should open the obstruction and remove the blockage. If the pain is due to weakness and insufficiency, we need to determine whether the qi and yang are too weak to move the qi or whether blood and yin are so insufficient they cannot nourish and fill the vessels. In the former case, we would boost the qi and so invigorate the yang. In the latter, we need to nourish the blood, which enriches the yin and fills the essence.

THE CAUSES AND MECHANISMS OF HEADACHES

Having explained the basic mechanisms of pain according to Chinese medicine, we will now turn to the specific causes and mechanisms of pain in the head, or headache. Pain may be caused by external pathogens or by poor function of one or more of the internal mechanisms of the body. These explanations are based on descriptions by Philippe Sionneau in his book *The Treatment of Disease in TCM* (see page 170).

CONTRACTION OF EXTERNAL EVILS

If our defensive qi is weak but external evils are strong, these external evils may take advantage of this relative vacuity and weakness to enter and invade the body. The most common external evils to invade the body and cause headache are wind, cold, dampness and heat. Normally wind combines with either cold and dampness or with heat. These external evils lodge in the channels and network vessels of the head and face and inhibit the free flow of the qi and blood in the affected area. As the free flow of qi and blood is affected, the result is pain.

INTERNAL DAMAGE

The liver, spleen and kidneys are the three viscera most commonly involved in this group of disease mechanisms; if they are damaged or functioning poorly, this may lead to pain.

Liver function

Every desire puts qi in motion. If a desire is unfulfilled, the qi of which it is an expression is blocked or thwarted and is not able to flow to its hoped-for destination or conclusion. Since it is the liver that is responsible for maintaining the coursing and discharging of the qi, such unfulfilled desires can damage the liver and impair its ability to function efficiently. In this case, the liver becomes depressed and the qi becomes stagnant. If the qi becomes stagnant, this leads it to back up and accumulate. The nature of the liver is inherently yang, so accumulated yang qi will tend to counterflow upwards like steam escaping from a pressure cooker. When this upwardly counterflowing liver qi or liver yang arrives in the 'bony box' of the head, it has nowhere else to go and no easy way out. It takes the place of the qi and blood that normally flow through the channels and network vessels of the head, inhibiting the qi and blood within the head, and so leading to pain.

Stress is often the result of wanting to do more than we have the time, energy, or wherewithal to accomplish. Stress is therefore often a compromise of the free flow of our desires. We are trying to rush somewhere to be on time but we get stuck in traffic. We are trying to get out a report for our boss, but our computer breaks down. We want to go to a football match with friends, but we have to stay late at work. The more stress we experience, the more liver depression qi stagnation we will have. Eventually, all this accumulated yang qi will have to go somewhere. If it goes upwards, it will usually cause a headache.

Kidney function

If, due to the ageing process, chronic disease, excessive sex, or too many drugs, kidney yang becomes vacuous and insufficient, there will not be enough yang qi to warm the body. Yang qi arises in the lower body and must ascend to the upper body to empower and warm the head. Cold is yin and constricting and congealing in nature. The qi and blood must be kept at a certain temperature for them to flow freely. If kidney yang is insufficient, the qi and blood flow in the brain may become inhibited or not free flowing. Thus there is pain in the head.

According to Chinese medical theory, the brain is the sea of marrow that is nourished and enriched by blood and essence. Blood and essence are both relatively yin. If, due to the ageing process or a number of other factors (such as prolonged excessive activity, overexertion, chronic disease, too much sex, overuse of drugs, alcohol, tobacco or caffeine) the yin blood is consumed, yin may fail to nourish the network vessels of the brain. These network vessels will fail to do their job, which is to transport the qi and blood. The free flow of the qi and blood in the brain is inhibited and the result is pain.

Spleen function

The spleen can cause at least three different sorts of headaches. The proper functioning of the spleen can be damaged by overwork, too little exercise, too much thinking and especially worry, or by improper diet. The spleen is easily damaged by eating too many chilled, uncooked foods, too many damp-producing foods, such as dairy products and oils and fats, and too much sugar. If the spleen becomes vacuous and weak, it may fail to move and transform body fluids. If these collect, they can transform into phlegm and dampness. If phlegm and dampness are wafted upwards in the body, they may lodge in the channels and network vessels of the head, obstructing and hindering the free flow of qi and blood.

Secondly, the spleen is the source of qi and blood transformation and engenderment. This means that it is mainly the spleen that is in charge of digestion of food and the creation of qi and blood out of the refined essence of food and liquids. So if the spleen is vacuous, so also may be the qi. If the qi becomes vacuous and weak, it may not be sufficient to move upwards to the head to move the blood and body fluids. Again, there is no free flow, and again, there is pain.

And lastly, if, for any reason, the spleen becomes vacuous and weak, it may not transform and engender sufficient blood. The blood is necessary to nourish the channels and vessels in the head. If these do not receive sufficient nourishment and enrichment, they may cease to function properly. Since their function is to promote the flow of qi and blood, once again, there is no free flow, and consequently there is pain.

Blood stasis

Static blood may result from local traumatic injury that severs the channels and vessels. The blood then flows outside the vessels and, as the blood can only flow when it is inside the vessels, it becomes static. Static blood then obstructs the flow of fresh blood, qi and body fluids. This results in pain. Static blood may also be caused by chronic disease affecting the free flow of the qi and body fluids. For instance, if there is stress, causing liver depression qi stagnation, and the qi remains stagnant for a long time, eventually this will result in blood stasis as well. As it is said in Chinese, 'If the qi moves, the blood moves. If the qi stops, the blood stops.' Similarly, if body fluids accumulate for any reason, because they are a yin substance, they will impede the free flow of yang qi. This means that eventually the qi will become stagnant and subsequently the blood as well.

Food retention

Food retention may also be involved with headaches. The retention of undigested or stagnant food in the stomach can aggravate liver depression qi stagnation. If we overeat or eat foods that are very hard to digest, stagnant food may be retained in the stomach. This yin stagnant food prevents the uninhibited, free flow of the qi. This then damages the liver and gives rise to, or aggravates, qi stagnation. If this accumulated, stagnant qi ascends and counterflows to the head, then the free flow of the qi and blood in the head will be compromised. No free flow equals pain.

According to Chinese medical theory, the mechanisms we have just described account for all headaches. Frequently, headaches are a combination of more than one of these mechanisms. For example, stress can cause a predisposition to liver depression qi stagnation and yang qi may be tending to vent itself upwards. The person may suffer from chronically tight shoulders and neck and a tendency to headaches. If they then suffer from a wind cold external invasion, i.e. catch a cold, this may constrict and congeal the qi and blood in the head sufficiently to trigger a headache. It is very common for liver depression due to stress to be complicated by blood vacuity due to a weak spleen, menstruation, overwork or a faulty diet. Another possibility could be for liver depression qi stagnation to become complicated by phlegm dampness due to poor spleen function, as a result of a poor diet and/or too little exercise.

ENLIGHTENMENT AND EMPOWERMENT

The beauty of Chinese medical theory is that it does identify in very real terms what the mechanisms are behind a headache. If you know that your headache is caused by phlegm dampness blocking the channels and network vessels in the head, then there are steps that can be taken to transform this phlegm and eliminate this dampness. More importantly, there are also steps you can take in order to prevent the creation of such phlegm and dampness. Chinese medicine is both enlightening and empowering, as it tells you why you are suffering from the headache and what steps you need to take to get rid of it and prevent its recurrence.

THE CHINESE MEDICAL TREATMENT OF HEADACHES

Fundamental to Chinese medicine is treatment based on what is called 'pattern discrimination'. Modern Western medicine bases its treatment on a disease diagnosis. This means that two patients diagnosed as suffering from the same disease will get the same treatment. Traditional Chinese medicine does take the patient's disease diagnosis into account, but the choice of treatment is not based on the disease so much as it is on the patient's 'pattern'. This aspect of Chinese medicine makes it holistic, safe and effective.

In order to explain the difference between a disease and a pattern, let us take the symptom of a headache as an example. All headaches by definition must involve some pain in the head. In modern Western medicine and other medical systems that prescribe primarily on the basis of a disease diagnosis, there is likely to be some sort of specific headache medication given. Headache sufferers can, however, be quite different – man or woman, young or old, overweight or thin, for example. The actual symptoms of the headache can also vary – the pain may be on the left or on the right side, it may be throbbing and continuous, or sharp but intermittent, etc. One sufferer could also have the following symptoms: indigestion, a tendency to loose stools, cold feet, red eyes, a dry mouth and desire for cold drinks, whilst another sufferer might have a wet, weeping, crusty skin rash with red borders, a tendency to hay fever, ringing in their ears and dizziness when they stand up. Whilst according to both Chinese medicine and modern Western medicine both people suffer from a headache, they also each suffer from a whole host of other complaints and so may have very different types of headaches. In Chinese medicine, the patient's pattern is made up from all these other signs and symptoms and further information. The pattern tries to describe the whole person as a unique individual. Treatment is designed to rebalance that entire pattern of imbalance as well as addressing the major complaint, symptom or disease. There is a saying in Chinese medicine: 'One disease, different treatments; different diseases, same treatment.'

This means that, in Chinese medicine, two patients with the same named disease diagnosis may receive different treatments if their Chinese medical patterns are different, while two patients diagnosed with different named diseases may receive the same treatment if their Chinese medical pattern is the same. The result always is that each person is treated individually.

Since every patient gets an individually tailored treatment to restore balance there are usually no unwanted side-effects. Side-effects come from forcing one part of the body to behave while causing an imbalance in another part. The treatment may have been appropriate to relieve part of the problem but it does not take into account the whole. This is like robbing Peter to pay Paul. The fact that Chinese medicine takes many aspects of a person into account and looks at the body as a single, unified whole means that a problem is treated without creating further imbalances.

PATTERN DISCRIMINATION OF HEADACHES

The following pattern discrimination for headaches comes from Philippe Sionneau's *The Treatment of Disease in TCM* (see page 170).

Wind cold

Symptoms: Recurrent pain that also affects the back of the neck and upper back; dislike of wind and cold, symptoms exacerbated by exposure to cold; thin, white tongue fur and a floating, tight pulse.[1] This sort of headache usually occurs with a common cold or flu, with airborne allergy attacks and the beginnings of sinusitis.

Therapeutic principles: Resolve the exterior, dispel wind, and scatter cold.

Wind heat

Symptoms: Headache accompanied by an exploding or splitting sensation; fever; dislike of wind; flushed red facial complexion; red eyes; a desire to drink; constipation; dark-coloured urine; a red tongue with yellow fur and a floating, rapid pulse. This type of headache is associated with common colds and the beginnings of sinusitis.

Therapeutic principles: Course wind and clear heat, open the network vessels and stop pain.

Wind dampness

Symptoms: Headache characterised by the sensation of something tight bound around the head; dizziness and heaviness of the head aggravated by damp, wet weather; chest oppression (a heavy sensation on the chest); epigastric fullness (full stomach); poor appetite; heavy limbs with lack of strength; scanty urination; loose stools; slimy, white tongue fur and a soggy, slippery pulse.

Therapeutic principles: Dispel wind and overcome dampness, open the network vessels and stop pain.

---

[1] Taking the pulse forms an important part of Chinese medical diagnosis. There are six different pulse positions on the radial artery of each wrist, giving information on the viscera, bowels and channels. There are 28 types of pulse quality, including floating, tight, soggy, slippery, wiry, etc.

Ascendant liver yang hyperactivity

Symptoms: Headache with dizziness or vertigo, commonly located in the temporal regions or top of the head; vexation (anxiety) and agitation; irritability; restless sleep; possible lateral costal (rib) pain; tinnitus; a flushed, red face; a bitter taste in the mouth; a red tongue with scanty or yellow fur and a wiry, forceful pulse. This pattern of headache may be found in migraine sufferers and people with hypertension (high blood pressure). It may also be found in those with chronic, recurrent, tension headaches.

Therapeutic principles: Level the liver, subdue yang and stop pain.

Exuberant liver fire

Symptoms: Headache with a distended (exploding) feeling in the head; headache often located at the top of the head; irritability; tinnitus; occasional pain and a sensation of heat in the lateral costal region; red eyes; dryness and a bitter taste in the mouth; dark-coloured urine; constipation; yellow tongue fur and a wiry, rapid pulse. This pattern may be seen in those with migraines, hypertension, sinusitis and trigeminal neuralgia (neuralgia affecting the largest cranial nerves).

Therapeutic principles: Clear the liver, drain fire and stop pain.

Kidney yin vacuity

Symptoms: Headache, characterised by an empty sensation in the head; vexatious (irritating) heat sensation; dry throat; dizziness; lower back and knee soreness and weakness; lassitude of the spirit; loss of semen; loss of sleep; a red tongue with scant fur and a fine, forceless pulse.

Therapeutic principles: Enrich yin and supplement the kidneys, stop pain.

Kidney yang vacuity

Symptoms: A dull headache and sometimes a cold sensation in the head; pain worsened by cold; dislike of cold; chilled limbs; a pale white facial complexion; a pale tongue and a deep and fine or deep and slow pulse

Therapeutic principles: Warm and supplement kidney yang, stop pain.

Blood vacuity

Symptoms: Dull headache with dizziness; heart palpitations; rubbing of the eyes and blurred vision; insomnia or poor sleep; apathy; a pale white facial complexion; pale lips, nails and tongue and a fine, weak pulse. Often, blood vacuity headaches occur after menstruation or when the sufferer is very fatigued; they may be complicated by liver yang hyperactivity.

Therapeutic principles: Nourish the blood and harmonise the network vessels, stop pain.

Qi vacuity

Symptoms: Dull headache with an empty sensation in the head that is worsened by overexertion; sweating on exertion; apathy; susceptibility to external pathogens; poor appetite; shortness of breath; loose stools; scanty, white tongue fur and a vacuous, forceless pulse. This pattern of headache may be due to fatigue or overwork.

Therapeutic principles: Supplement the centre and boost the qi, stop pain.

Damp phlegm

Symptoms: Headache with dizziness; sensation of fullness in the stomach; chest oppression; a possible heavy sensation in the body; vomiting of phlegmy saliva; poor appetite; apathy; slimy, white tongue fur and a wiry, slippery pulse.

Therapeutic principles: Fortify the spleen and transform phlegm, open the network vessels and stop pain.

Blood stasis

Symptoms: Obstinate, pricking headache with fixed location with a history of trauma (injury) or as a result of chronic disease; a purple tongue with scant, white fur and a fine and choppy, or deep and choppy pulse. Blood stasis may complicate a number of these other patterns. This is because blood stasis tends to occur whenever there is chronic or long-lasting disease. If you have had severe, recurrent headaches for a long time, look for signs and symptoms of blood stasis along with the symptoms of other patterns.

Therapeutic principles: Quicken the blood and transform stasis, move the qi and stop pain.

Food retention

Symptoms: Headache; fullness in the chest and stomach; aversion to food; acid regurgitation; belching of putrid wind; thick, slimy tongue fur and a wiry pulse. Food retention headaches are usually associated with a particular episode of eating and drinking too much. Food stagnation is not usually associated with chronic headaches.

Therapeutic principles: Disperse food and abduct stagnation.

You can see from the above pattern descriptions with their treatment principles that each different pattern requires different treatment principles to return the person back into balance. This means that there is no single headache remedy in Chinese medicine, and a remedy that is beneficial for one pattern might actually make a person with a different pattern worse.

Most chronic headaches are associated with liver yang hyperactivity, kidney yin vacuity, blood vacuity, qi vacuity and phlegm dampness. In clinical practice, most patients with chronic headaches have a combination of more than one pattern. For example, in women with menstrual migraine headaches, it is not unusual to find liver yang hyperactivity with blood vacuity and blood stasis. Another common menstrual migraine pattern is qi and blood vacuity with blood stasis. In heavy-set, overweight men and women, it is not unusual to find a combination of liver yang hyperactivity with phlegm and dampness. In practice, the simple traditional Chinese medicine patterns we have discussed do have to be modified to fit patients individually.

HOW THE SYSTEM WORKS IN REAL LIFE

Using all this information on the theory of Chinese medicine and the patterns and their mechanisms of headache, let us now see how a practitioner of Chinese medicine makes this system work in practice.

Take Jean, for example, whom we introduced at the beginning of this book. She has experienced migraine headaches on and off since she was about 13. Usually Jean's migraines occur at the onset of her menstrual periods. They can also occur if she is under a lot of stress or if she eats peanuts or chocolate. Her migraines are preceded by a visual aura and tingling and numbness on her face and hands. The pain is pounding and always located on the left side. During an attack, she cannot bear any light or sound. At some point in an attack, Jean becomes so nauseous she vomits and often also experiences diarrhoea. After this, she can usually fall asleep. When Jean wakes up, the headache is gone. In terms of menstruation, Jean reports that she does have premenstrual stress (PMS). She becomes irritable and is easily angered for a week before each menses. Her breasts become swollen and sore and her nipples are especially sensitive during that same time.

Her tongue appears puffy. It is generally a bit paler than normal, but the tip and left edge are redder than normal. Her pulse is bowstring, fine and a bit rapid. It also feels soggy over her wrist bone on the right side.

ANALYSIS OF JEAN'S SYMPTOMS

Jean's premenstrual irritability, her swollen, sore breasts and her hypersensitive nipples all point towards liver depression qi stagnation. This is corroborated by her bowstring pulse. In Jean's case, there is also blood vacuity. We know this because her tongue is generally paler than normal and her pulse is also fine. This blood vacuity is due to spleen weakness. We diagnose this because of the slightly puffy tongue and the soggy pulse over the right wrist bone, the pulse position corresponding to the spleen. Jean's liver depression qi stagnation gets worse in the week before her menses arrive because the body's blood collects in the uterus for expulsion with the period. If the blood is vacuous and insufficient, this does not leave enough for it to perform its proper functions in the rest of the body. Since the liver can only function if it receives blood to nourish it, the liver's coursing and discharging becomes even more dysfunctional before the period. This is why Jean gets PMS and why her migraines are mostly associated with her periods. The fact that she gets her migraines on the left side also confirms this, as the left side of the body corresponds to the blood.

Jean's liver depression qi stagnation gets worse before her menses and in her case the stagnant qi tends to transform into heat or hyperactive yang. This is confirmed by the rapid pulse and the red tongue tip and left-side pain, the left side also corresponding to the liver. This accumulated liver qi that has transformed into hyperactive liver yang has to go somewhere, so it counterflows upwards along the yang channel connected to the liver, the gall bladder and triple burner channels. These two channels traverse the sides of the head.

Some of the liver qi also vents horizontally to attack the stomach and spleen. When the liver attacks the stomach, there is nausea and even vomiting. If the liver qi attacks the spleen, there may be diarrhoea. If there is vomiting or diarrhoea, however, a lot of qi is discharged with the vomit and stools. This is like releasing the safety valve on a pressure cooker. The liver qi is vented outside the body and it does not counterflow upwards into the head. Hence, the headache subsides. As Jean has also vented and lost a lot of qi, she falls asleep.

The tingling around the mouth and hands shows that there is blood vacuity, and also that the qi is starting to move chaotically in the body. The visual aura and photophobia (aversion to light) both have to do with the liver. The eyes are the portals of the liver, according to Chinese medicine, so they can see only when they receive sufficient blood to nourish them. The flashing lights, dazzling lines, etc., that many migraine sufferers experience, are manifestations of the yang qi flooding the head from the liver. The fact that the patient cannot stand any outside light or noise has to do with both of these stimuli being types of yang qi entering the head from outside. There is already far too much yang qi pounding inside Jean's head to tolerate any more entering from outside.

The fact that nuts and chocolate can both sometimes trigger a migraine attack is due to their being oily, fatty foods. Oil and fat are damp and hot, as is hyperactivity of liver yang, so they exacerbate the situation. Additionally, cocoa is considered hot and particularly inflames an aspect of heat in the body that relates to liver yang.

If we add all this information up, we know that there is liver depression transforming into liver yang hyperactivity, which then counterflows upwards into the head. This liver depression is aggravated by blood vacuity, which in turn is aggravated by the menstrual cycle because the blood is sent downwards to the uterus from the premenstruum through the period itself.

HOW JEAN'S HEADACHE IS TREATED

Jean's case is characterised by two phases. There the 'normal' time between migraine attacks and there are the attacks themselves. Between attacks, the practitioner will attempt to course Jean's liver and rectify her qi, supplement her spleen and nourish her blood. Since the liver yang hyperactivity causing the migraines transforms from liver depression qi stagnation and is aggravated by blood vacuity in turn due to spleen vacuity, these principles will form the basis of the treatment towards preventing further occurrences of Jean's migraines by treating the root mechanisms of her head pain.

During the attacks themselves, the treatment principles are to clear liver heat, reverse upward counterflow, subdue yang and nourish the blood. Jean's Chinese medical treatment is divided into two phases. Phase one is designed to treat the underlying root mechanisms of Jean's migraines during the time between attacks. Phase two is designed to stop or prevent the migraines during the time they are most likely to occur, during the premenstrual period and the menses.

Once the practitioner has stated the treatment principles necessary for re-establishing balance within the patient, then anything that works to accomplish these principles will be beneficial for the patient. Using these principles, there are now several methods of treatment to choose from. The two main treatment methods are acupuncture and Chinese herbal medicine. It is also possible that the practitioner will make recommendations on appropriate diet and lifestyle changes.

Since Chinese herbal medicine is one of the main methods of treatment, let's look at how a prescription is crafted for Jean. The first treatment principles stated for Jean were to course the liver and rectify the qi, supplement the spleen and nourish the blood, so we know that we should select our guiding formula from the category of formulae designed to harmonise the liver and spleen. Depending on the textbook, there are 22–28 main categories of formulae in Chinese medicine, each category correlated to a main treatment principle. The category of harmonising the liver and spleen is part of a broader category of harmonising formulae that are used to treat patterns that involve complex processes in different levels and organs of the body, as well as the simultaneous presence of hot and cold

Under this category of formulae, there is one very well known formula, *Xiao Yao Wan* (Rambling Powder) which addresses all of the above treatment principles we have stated are necessary. This formula can be used for a wide variety of complaints characterised by both liver depression qi stagnation and spleen vacuity giving rise to blood vacuity. This basic prescription would then be modified to address the specific patient's complaints more effectively.

The standard formula consists of:

Radix Bupleuri *(Chai Hu)*
Radix Albus Paeoniae Lactiflorae *(Bai Shao)*
Radix Angelicae Sinensis *(Dang Gui)*
Rhizoma Atractylodis Macrocephalae *(Bai Zhu)*
Sclerotium Poriae Cocos *(Fu Ling)*
Herba Menthae Haplocalycis *(Bo He)*
Mix-fried Radix Glycyrrhizae *(Gan Cao)*
Uncooked Rhizoma Zingiberis *(Sheng Jiang)*

Bupleurum courses the liver, rectifies the qi, and resolves depression. Paeonia and Angelica both nourish the blood and, by doing so, also soften and harmonise the liver. Atractylodes and Poria supplement the spleen so it can transform and engender the blood. Additionally, Poria leads any yang qi or evil heat downwards in the body rather than up. Mentha helps Bupleurum course the liver and resolve depression. Both are somewhat cooling, so they keep liver depression from transforming into depressive heat or hyperactive yang. Uncooked Zingiber (ginger) assists Bupleurum in moving the qi, while it assists Atractylodes and Poria in getting rid of any dampness that may hinder the functioning of the spleen. Finally, Glycyrrhiza (liquorice) supplements the spleen, nourishes heart blood and calms the spirit, whilst also harmonising all the other ingredients into a cohesive, healthful whole.

This formula might be given to Jean from the time of ovulation onwards till day 21 or the onset of any premenstrual symptoms. Usually, a formula such as this would be taken two to three times each day. The herbs would be soaked in water and then boiled for 30–45 minutes into a very strong infusion or tea.

During the premenstruum itself, the practitioner would probably change Jean's prescription to a different formula, designed specifically for liver yang hyperactivity. One such formula is *Tian Ma Gou Teng Yin* (Gastrodia and Uncaria Drink). Its ingredients include:

Rhizoma Gastrodiae Elatae *(Tian Ma)*
Ramulus Uncariae Cum Uncis *(Gou Teng)*
Concha Haliotidis *(Shi Jue Ming)*
Ramulus Loranthi Seu Visci *(Sang Ji Sheng)*
Cortex Eucommiae Ulmoidis *(Du Zhong)*
Radix Cyathulae *(Chuan Niu Xi)*
Fructus Gardeniae Jasminoidis *(Shan Zhi Zi)*
Radix Scutellariae Baicalensis *(Huang Qin)*
Herba Leonuri Heterophylli *(Yi Mu Cao)*
Caulis Polygoni Multiflori *(Ye Jiao Teng)*
Sclerotium Poriae Cocos *(Fu Ling)*

Within this formula, Gastrodia and Uncaria both level liver wind, while Uncaria clears liver heat. Liver wind means chaotically counterflowing liver qi ascending to the head and running around in the skin. Loranthus and Eucommia both nourish the blood and supplement the kidneys. The kidneys are the mother of the liver and the blood is the mother of qi.

Supplementing the blood and kidneys helps to control liver yang. Cyathula leads the qi to move downwards, not up, as does Poria, and Gardenia and Scutellaria both clear heat from the liver. Leonurus quickens the blood and transforms stasis. If there is long-term liver depression qi stagnation, there is often at least an element of blood stasis. Caulis Polygoni Multiflori courses the liver and resolves depression, nourishes the heart and quiets the spirit. As the headache occurs on the side of the head and in order to make this formula more powerful in moving the qi and blood in the head, we might add some Radix Ligustici Wallichii *(Chuan Xiong)* to the above prescription.

The ingredients in these two formulae may also be taken as a dried, powdered extract. Such extracts are manufactured by several Taiwanese and Japanese companies. Although these extracts are not, in my experience, as powerful as the freshly decocted teas, they are easier to take. Many standard formulae also come as ready-made pills. Pills cannot, however, be modified. If their ingredients match the patient's requirements, then they are quite acceptable, but if the formula needs modifications, then teas or powders where individual ingredients can be added and subtracted are better.

In exactly the same way, based on Jean's pattern discrimination and treatment principles, the practitioner of Chinese medicine could create an individual acupuncture treatment plan and an accompanying dietary and lifestyle plan. However, we will discuss each of these later in their own chapters.

In a woman with Jean's Chinese pattern discrimination and long history of migraines, we can expect that she will need to take the Chinese herbal medicine for at least three months or menstrual cycles. After that, she may want to go back on one or the other of these formulae whenever she is under special stress. However, the main preventive treatment lies in identifying the dietary and lifestyle factors that bring on the problem in the first place and then modifying or avoiding these. Migraines are not something that can be cured once and for all, like measles. Jean will still have to be careful at least until she passes through the menopause. She will, however, learn what she can do for herself, and she also will know that there is Chinese medicine that can help support her when times get rough and stress is unavoidable.

CHINESE HERBAL MEDICINE AND HEADACHES

As we have seen from Jean's case, there is no single Chinese herb or even a single herbal formula that will work for all headache sufferers. Chinese medicinals are prescribed based on a person's pattern discrimination, and are specifically selected to suit the individual and their particular symptoms.

Since most headaches are a combination of different Chinese patterns and disease mechanisms, Chinese medicine never treats headaches with a single herb given on its own. Chinese herbal medicine is based on rebalancing patterns, and patterns in real-life patients almost always have more than a single element. Chinese herbalists almost always prescribe herbs in multi-ingredient formulae. Such formulae may have anywhere between four and 20 ingredients. If a practitioner of Chinese medicine reads a prescription given by another practitioner, they will be able to tell you not only what the patient's pattern discrimination was but also what the likely signs and symptoms were. In creating a herbal formula, the practitioner of Chinese medicine does not just combine several herbs that are reputed to be 'good for headaches'. Rather, a formula is carefully crafted with ingredients to rebalance every aspect of the patient's body–mind.

GETTING THE RIGHT HERBAL MEDICINE TREATMENT FOR YOURSELF

Chinese herbal medicine has become increasingly popular in the West, particularly in the UK. It does, however, require a high level of study as it is quite complex and I strongly recommend that you seek professional advice. As well as the signs and symptoms of an illness, a practitioner of Chinese medicine will take into account additional information, such as tongue and pulse diagnosis (see footnote on page 48), in order to decide which herbs are appropriate. These skills require experience and training and are beyond the scope of this book. This means that the self-prescribing of Chinese herbs is really not something for the layperson to attempt, especially if unsupervised. As a layperson, it is unlikely that you will be able to obtain Chinese herbs without a prescription from a qualified practitioner in the UK, as reputable suppliers don't generally sell directly to the public. Chinese herbal medicines can be very powerful; just as they have the power to heal, they can also do damage if incorrectly used. You will find suggestions on how to find a qualified professional Chinese medical practitioner near you on pages 147–50.

CHINESE PATENT MEDICINES

The remainder of this chapter will focus on what are commonly known as Chinese herbal patent remedies or 'patents'. These are herbal remedies that have been used for many years, often for centuries, and therefore have a tried-and-tested track record for treating illness. In some countries they may be available over the counter in a health food shop or Chinese herb specialist shop, but I strongly recommend that you do not take them unsupervised. I have included them here as they demonstrate how Chinese herbal medicine treats headaches. Even an individually tailored herbal medicine prescription will often include the herbs presented in these formulae.

On pages 48–51, I gave the signs and symptoms of the 12 basic patterns associated with headaches. These are:

1. Wind cold
2. Wind heat

3. Wind dampness
4. Hyperactivity of ascendant liver yang
5. Exuberant liver fire
6. Kidney yin vacuity
7. Kidney yang vacuity
8. Blood vacuity
9. Qi vacuity
10. Damp phlegm
11. Blood stasis
12. Food retention

As each patent remedy is discussed, we will give details of the pattern and signs and symptoms for which it is appropriate.

Chuan Xiong Cha Tiao Wan

The name of this medicine translates as Ligusticum and Tea Mixed Pills. It is a specific remedy for wind cold headache. Since it contains a number of ingredients that move the qi and quicken the blood in the various channels that traverse the head and face, it can be used for first-aid purposes for most replete kinds of head and face pain. This formula also treats wind damp headache. Its ingredients include:

Radix Ligustici Wallichii *(Chuan Xiong)*
Radix Et Rhizoma Notopterygii *(Qiang Huo)*
Radix Angelicae Dahuricae *(Bai Zhi)*
Herba Asari Cum Radice *(Xi Xin)*
Herba Seu Flos Schizonepetae Tenuifoliae *(Jing Jie Sui)*
Radix Ledebouriellae Divaricatae *(Fang Feng)*
Herba Menthae Haplocalycis *(Bo He)*
Radix Glycyrrhizae *(Gan Cao)*
Folium Camilliae Chinensis *(Cha Ye)*

Notopterygium, Angelica, Schizonepeta, Ledebouriella, Mentha and Camillia all resolve the exterior and scatter wind.

The first four of these are warm in nature and also scatter cold. The last two are cool in nature and clear heat. Asarum is quite warm and enters the smallest network vessels in order to quicken the blood. Ligusticum also quickens the blood, especially in the head. Glycyrrhiza harmonises all the ingredients in the formula and helps to minimise any side-effects, particularly those of the digestive system.

These pills can be taken in combination with some of the other Chinese patent medicines corresponding to other patterns designed specifically to help to treat symptoms of pain in the head more effectively. These pills should not be used with yin or blood vacuity, since the ingredients in this formula are very drying and tend to consume and damage blood and yin in those with a yin vacuous bodily constitution.

Sang Ju Yin

This formula, which translates as Morus and Chrysanthemum Drink, is the standard guiding formula for wind heat common cold and cough where there is also an element of dryness. It also includes at least two ingredients for treating hot-natured headaches. The ingredients include:

Folium Mori Albi *(Sang Ye)*
Flos Chrysanthemi Morifolii *(Ju Hua)*
Herba Menthae Haplocalycis *(Bo He)*
Semen Pruni Armeniacae *(Xing Ren)*
Radix Platycodi Grandiflori *(Jie Geng)*
Fructus Forsythiae Suspensae *(Lian Qiao)*
Rhizoma Phragmitis Communis *(Lu Gen)*
Radix Glycyrrhizae *(Gan Cao)*

Morus and Chrysanthemum both clear heat from the head, face and eyes. They resolve the exterior and effuse wind while also clearing heat. Externally invading wind heat often stirs up or compounds any existing liver heat. Both these two medicinals address not only wind heat but also liver heat and yang hyperactivity. They are assisted by Mentha, which also resolves the exterior and clears both exterior and liver heat. Armeniaca transforms phlegm, moistens dryness and stops coughing. Platycodon also transforms phlegm and stops coughing. Forsythia resolves the exterior and clears heat. Phragmites engenders or creates stomach and intestinal fluids. Glycyrrhiza harmonises the entire formula whilst also clearing some heat. Since Armeniaca and Phragmites both enrich the stomach and engender fluids in the bowels, they promote the free flow of the stools. (Constipation is very likely in this pattern.) If the bowels move downwards, then this relieves pressure and pain in the head. In this instance, having an enema can also help relieve the headache as well as the other symptoms of this pattern.

Xin Yi Wan
Called Magnolia Flower Pills in English, these pills are especially effective for relieving blocked nasal passages and sinus pressure due to wind damp invasion. The ingredients are:

Flos Magnoliae Lilleflorae *(Xin Yi)*
Rhizoma Atractylodis Macrocephalae *(Bai Zhu)*
Radix Ledebouriellae Divaricatae *(Fang Feng)*
Herba Asari Cum Radice *(Xi Xin)*
Radix Et Rhizoma Notopterygii *(Qiang Huo)*
Radix Et Rhizoma Ligustici Sinensis *(Gao Ben)*
Radix Ligustici Wallichii *(Chuan Xiong)*
Rhizoma Cimicifugae *(Sheng Ma)*
Caulis Akebiae *(Mu Tong)*
Radix Glycyrrhizae *(Gan Cao)*

Bi Yan Pian

These pills are called Rhinitis Tablets in English. They are for acute or chronic rhinitis, sinusitis with runny nose and large amounts of thick, yellow, pussy discharge, stuffy nose, hay fever and the headache that often accompanies such symptoms. In terms of Chinese pattern discrimination, these tablets treat wind heat. The ingredients are:

Fructus Xanthii Sibirici *(Cang Er Zi)*
Flos Magnoliae Lilleflorae *(Xin Yi)*
Radix Glycyrrhizae *(Gan Cao)*
Cortex Phellodendri *(Huang Bai)*
Radix Platycodi Grandiflori *(Jie Geng)*
Fructus Schisandrae Chinensis *(Wu Wei Zi)*
Fructus Forsythiae Suspensae *(Lian Qiao)*
Radix Angelicae Dahuricae *(Bai Zhi)*
Rhizoma Anemarrhenae Aspheloidis *(Zhi Mu)*
Flos Chrysanthemi Indici *(Ye Ju Hua)*
Radix Ledebouriellae Divaricatae *(Fang Feng)*
Herba Seu Flos Schizonepetae Tenuifoliae *(Jing Jie Sui)*

It is particularly important not to exceed the recommended dosage as stated on the packaging. The Chung Lian brand of this formula contains acetaminophen.

Huo Xiang Zheng Qi Wan

The name of these pills translates as Agastaches Correct the Qi Pills. They are based on a very old and very well known formula for 'summerheat' flu. This means that they treat wind damp heat. The symptoms of this are fever, chills, headache, upper abdominal distention, abdominal pain, nausea, vomiting, flatulence and either diarrhoea or sticky, incomplete stools. The tongue fur is white and slimy. The ingredients in this formula include:

Herba Agastachis Seu Pogostemi *(Huo Xiang)*
Radix Angelicae Dahuricae *(Bai Zhi)*
Pericarpium Arecae Catechu *(Da Fu Pi)*
Folium Perillae Frutescentis *(Zi Su Ye)*
Sclerotium Poriae Cocos *(Fu Ling)*
Rhizoma Atractylodis Macrocephalae *(Bai Zhu)*
Cortex Magnoliae Officinalis *(Hou Po)*
Radix Platycodi Grandiflori *(Jie Geng)*
Pericarpium Citri Reticulatae *(Chen Pi)*
Radix Glycyrrhizae *(Gan Cao)*

Xiao Yao Wan (also spelt *Hsiao Yao Wan*)

Xiao Yao Wan is one of the most common Chinese herbal formulae prescribed. Its Chinese name has been translated as Free and Easy Pills, Rambling Pills, Relaxed Wanderer Pills and several other versions of this same idea of promoting a freer and smoother, more relaxed flow. As a patent medicine, this formula comes as pills, and there are both Chinese-made and American-made versions of this formula available. When marketed as a dried, powdered extract, this formula is sold under the name of Bupleurum and Tangkuei Formula.

The ingredients in this formula are:

Radix Bupleuri *(Chai Hu)*
Radix Angelicae Sinensis *(Dang Gui)*
Radix Albus Paeoniae Lactiflorae *(Bai Shao)*
Rhizoma Atractylodis Macrocephalae *(Bai Zhu)*
Sclerotium Poriae Cocos *(Fu Ling)*
Mix-fried Radix Glycyrrhizae *(Gan Cao)*
Herba Menthae Haplocalycis *(Bo He)*
Uncooked Rhizoma Zingiberis *(Sheng Jiang)*

This formula treats the pattern of liver depression qi stagnation complicated by blood vacuity and spleen weakness with possible dampness as well. Bupleurum courses the liver and rectifies the qi. It is aided in this by Mentha. Angelica and Paeonia nourish the blood and soften and harmonise the liver. Atractylodes and Poria fortify the spleen and eliminate dampness. Mix-fried Glycyrrhiza aids these two in fortifying the spleen and supplementing the liver, while uncooked Zingiber aids in both promoting and regulating the qi flow and eliminating dampness.

Liver depression qi stagnation typically precedes ascendant liver yang hyperactivity, which is one of the patterns of headache described by Philippe Sionneau earlier. This formula can be taken in order to prevent the tendency for liver depression to transform into liver heat or hyperactivity. The symptoms of this pattern include chest and rib-side distension and pain, irritability, chest oppression, emotional depression, a tendency to sigh, premenstrual breast distension and soreness, possible premenstrual lower abdominal distension and cramping, a normal or slightly dark tongue with a thin, white coating and a bowstring pulse.

As Bupleurum is very drying and has an upbearing effect, if after taking these pills at the dose recommended on the packaging you notice any side-effects, then stop immediately and seek professional advice. The side-effects from this formula might include nervousness, irritability, a dry mouth and increased thirst, provocation or worsening of headaches and red, dry eyes. The appearance of side-effects such as these would show that this formula, at least without modification, is not right for you. Although it may be doing you some good, it is also causing some harm. Chinese medicine is meant to cure without side-effects, and as long as the prescription matches your pattern there should not be any.

Dan Zhi Xiao Yao Wan
Dan Zhi Xiao Yao Wan or Moutan and Gardenia Rambling Pills is a modification of the above formula, which also comes as a

patent medicine in the form of pills. When marketed as a dried, powdered extract, this formula is called Bupleurum and Peony Formula. It is meant to treat the pattern of liver depression transforming into heat with spleen vacuity and possible blood vacuity and/or dampness. The ingredients in this formula are the same as the previous formula with the addition of two other herbs:

Cortex Radicis Moutan *(Dan Pi)*
Fructus Gardeniae Jasminoidis *(Shan Zhi Zi)*

These two ingredients clear heat and resolve depression. In addition, Moutan quickens the blood, dispels stasis and is effective in clearing heat specifically from the blood.

Basically, the signs and symptoms of the pattern for which this formula is designed are the same as those for *Xiao Yao Wan* (see page 67) plus signs and symptoms of depressive heat. These might include a reddish tongue with slightly yellow fur, a bowstring and rapid pulse, a bitter taste in the mouth and increased irritability. It is my experience that this pattern may be present especially in women with menstrual migraines or one-sided headaches.

Tian Ma Gou Teng Wan

The name of these pills translates as Gastrodia and Uncaria Pills. They are the standard textbook formula for ascendant hyperactivity of liver yang. Their ingredients are:

Rhizoma Gastrodiae Elatae *(Tian Ma)*
Ramulus Uncariae Cum Uncis *(Gou Teng)*
Concha Haliotidis *(Shi Jue Ming)*
Ramulus Loranthi Seu Visci *(Sang Ji Sheng)*
Cortex Eucommiae Ulmoidis *(Du Zhong)*
Fructus Gardeniae Jasminoidis *(Shan Zhi Zi)*
Radix Scutellariae Baicalensis *(Huang Qin)*

Radix Cyathulae *(Chuan Niu Xi)*
Herba Leonuri Heterophylli *(Yi Mu Cao)*
Caulis Polygoni Multiflori *(Ye Jiao Teng)*
Sclerotium Poriae Cocos *(Fu Ling)*

I have already described the functions of each of these medicinals in the previous chapter when discussing Jean's Chinese medicinal treatment. These pills work best when taken to prevent a liver yang headache as opposed to trying to relieve a fully developed migraine or cluster headache.

Huang Lian Shang Qing Pian (also spelt **Huang Lian Shang Ching Pian**)
These pills treat headache due to wind heat, hyperactivity of liver yang, and/or liver fire. Their name means Coptis Clear the Upper Tablets, the 'upper' here referring to the head. The ingredients are:

Rhizoma Coptidis Chinensis *(Huang Lian)*
Radix Ligustici Wallichii *(Chuan Xiong)*
Herba Seu Flos Schizonepetae Tenuifoliae *(Jing Jie Sui)*
Radix Ledebouriellae Divaricatae *(Fang Feng)*
Radix Scutellariae Baicalensis *(Huang Qin)*
Radix Platycodi Grandiflori *(Jie Geng)*
Gypsum Fibrosum *(Shi Gao)*
Flos Chrysanthemi Indici *(Ye Ju Hua)*
Radix Angelicae Dahuricae *(Bai Zhi)*
Radix Glycyrrhizae *(Gan Cao)*
Radix Et Rhizoma Rhei *(Da Huang)*
Fructus Viticis *(Man Jing Zi)*
Fructus Forsythiae Suspensae *(Lian Qiao)*
Flos Inulae *(Xuan Fu Hua)*
Cortex Phellodendri *(Huang Bai)*
Herba Menthae Haplocalycis *(Bo He)*
Fructus Gardeniae Jasminoidis *(Shan Zhi Zi)*

These pills are best used if there is also constipation. They should not be used when there is diarrhoea. If they cause diarrhoea, they should be stopped. Pregnant women should not take this remedy. It is not meant for long-term usage since it is extremely draining.

Long Dan Xie Gan Wan

Long dan means dragon gall. This is the literal translation of the name of the main ingredient in this formula, Gentiana. *Xie Gan* means drain the liver, while *wan* simply means pills. This formula is the textbook standard formula for liver fire. The symptoms of liver fire have been given earlier. The ingredients in this formula are:

Radix Gentianae Scabrae *(Long Dan Cao)*
Fructus Gardeniae Jasminoidis *(Shan Zhi Zi)*
Radix Scutellariae Baicalensis *(Huang Qin)*
Radix Bupleuri *(Chai Hu)*
Caulis Akebiae *(Mu Tong)*
Semen Plantaginis *(Che Qian Zi)*
Rhizoma Alisma *(Ze Xie)*
Uncooked Radix Rehmanniae *(Sheng Di)*
Extremitas Radicis Angelicae Sinensis *(Dang Gui Wei)*
Radix Glycyrrhizae *(Gan Cao)*

The ingredients in this formula are very bitter and cold and can, therefore, easily damage the spleen and stomach. This formula should only be taken for a few days. Once the signs of liver fire have abated, its use should be discontinued. If you develop diarrhoea while taking this formula, stop and seek advice from a practitioner. This formula is not meant for long-term usage, but for the treatment of acute conditions.

Gui Pi Wan (also spelt *Kuei Pi Wan*)

Gui means to return or restore, *pi* means the spleen, and *wan* means pills. So, the name of these pills translates as Restore the Spleen Pills. When sold as a dried, powdered extract, this formula is called Ginseng and Longan Combination. These pills not only supplement the spleen qi but also nourish heart blood and calm the heart spirit. They are the textbook guiding formula for the pattern of heart–spleen dual vacuity. In this pattern, there are symptoms of spleen qi vacuity, such as fatigue, poor appetite and cold hands and feet, plus symptoms of heart blood vacuity, such as a pale tongue, heart palpitations and insomnia. This formula is also the standard one for treating heavy or abnormal bleeding, such as heavy menstrual bleeding, due to the spleen not containing and restraining the blood within its vessels. This patent medicine can be combined with *Xiao Yao Wan* (see page 67) when there is liver depression qi stagnation complicated by heart blood and spleen qi vacuity. It is the most effective Chinese patent medicine for blood vacuity headaches. Its ingredients are:

Radix Astragali Membranacei *(Huang Qi)*
Radix Codonopsitis Pilosulae *(Dang Shen)*
Rhizoma Atractylodis Macrocephalae *(Bai Zhu)*
Sclerotium Parardicis Poriae Cocos *(Fu Shen)*
Mix-fried Radix Glycyrrhizae *(Gan Cao)*
Radix Angelicae Sinensis *(Dang Gui)*
Semen Zizyphi Spinosae *(Suan Zao Ren)*
Arillus Euphoriae Longanae *(Long Yan Rou)*
Radix Polygalae Tenuifoliae *(Yuan Zhi)*
Radix Auklandiae Lappae *(Mu Xiang)*

Bai Zi Yang Xin Wan

This is another popular Chinese patent pill for a combination of spleen qi vacuity and heart blood vacuity. Its name means Biota Nourish the Heart Pills. They are especially effective when headaches are accompanied by insomnia. The ingredients are:

Semen Biotae Orientalis *(Bai Zi Ren)*
Fructus Lycii Chinensis *(Gou Qi Zi)*
Radix Scrophulariae Ningpoensis *(Xuan Shen)*
Uncooked Radix Rehmanniae *(Sheng Di)*
Tuber Ophiopogonis Japonici *(Mai Dong)*
Radix Angelicae Sinensis *(Dang Gui)*
Sclerotium Poriae Cocos *(Fu Ling)*
Rhizoma Acori Graminei *(Shi Chang Pu)*
Radix Glycyrrhizae *(Gan Cao)*

Er Chen Wan

Er Chen Wan means Two Aged (Ingredients) Pills, because two of its main ingredients are aged before using. When sold as a dried, powdered extract, this formula is called Citrus and Pinellia Combination. It is used to transform phlegm and eliminate dampness and it can be added to virtually any other Chinese patent medicine when there is a heavy component of phlegm and dampness. Its ingredients are:

Rhizoma Pinelliae Ternatae *(Ban Xia)*
Sclerotium Poriae Cocos *(Fu Ling)*
Mix-fried Radix Glycyrrhizae *(Gan Cao)*
Pericarpium Citri Reticulatae *(Chen Pi)*
Uncooked Rhizoma Zingiberis *(Sheng Jiang)*

All these medicinals either transform phlegm or eliminate dampness.

Liu Wei Di Huang Wan

This formula, whose name means Six Flavours Rehmannia Pills, nourishes liver blood and kidney yin. It is the primary formula to treat symptoms of yin vacuity. Its ingredients are:

Cooked Radix Rehmanniae *(Shu Di)*
Fructus Corni Officinalis *(Shan Zhu Yu)*
Radix Dioscoreae Oppositae *(Shan Yao)*
Rhizoma Alismatis *(Ze Xie)*
Sclerotium Poriae Cocos *(Fu Ling)*
Cortex Radicis Moutan *(Dan Pi)*

In some people, Rehmannia can cause diarrhoea. If this happens, then stop taking the formula immediately.

If there is liver yang hyperactivity but with more pronounced underlying yin vacuity, then these pills can be combined with *Tian Ma Gou Teng Wan* (see page 69). If there are signs and symptoms of vacuity heat, such as flushed cheeks in the afternoon, low-grade fever and/or night sweats, then another formula should be used instead. It is made by adding two more ingredients to the above:

Rhizoma Anemarrhenae Aspheloidis *(Zhi Mu)*
Cortex Phellodendri *(Huang Bai)*

This combination is then called *Zhi Bai Di Huang Wan*, meaning Anemarrhena and Phellodendron Rehmannia Pills.

An Shen Bu Xin Wan
The name of this pill translates as Quiet the Spirit and Supplement the Heart Pills. They can be used to treat headache due to yin vacuity. These pills can be used instead of *Liu Wei Di Huang Wan* (above) if it causes diarrhoea. The ingredients are:

Concha Margaritiferae *(Zhen Zhu Mu)*
Caulis Polygoni Multiflori *(Ye Jiao Teng)*
Fructus Ligustri Lucidi *(Nu Zhen Zi)*
Herba Ecliptae Prostratae *(Han Lian Cao)*
Radix Salviae Miltiorrhizae *(Dan Shen)*

Cortex Albizziae Julibrissin *(He Huan Pi)*
Semen Cuscutae Chinensis *(Tu Si Zi)*
Fructus Schisandrae Chinensis *(Wu Wei Zi)*
Rhizoma Acori Graminei *(Shi Chang Pu)*

You Gui Wan

The name of these pills translates as Restore the Right Pills. This is because kidney yang is often referred to as the right kidney. This formula, therefore, is for the treatment of kidney yang vacuity headache. If there are cold symptoms present, such as cold feet, chilly, weak lower back, copious, clear, night-time urination or decreased sexual desire, you should not use this formula. You should also suspend its use if it produces symptoms of evil heat. These might include sores on the tongue or in the mouth, sore throat, fever and flu-like symptoms. This formula's ingredients are:

Cooked Radix Rehmanniae *(Shu Di)*
Radix Lateralis Praeparatus Aconiti Carmichaeli *(Fu Zi)*
Cortex Cinnamomi Cassiae *(Rou Gui)*
Fructus Corni Officinalis *(Shan Zhu Yu)*
Fructus Lycii Chinensis *(Wu Wei Zi)*
Radix Dioscoreae Oppositae *(Shan Yao)*
Cortex Eucommiae Ulmoidis *(Du Zhong)*
Radix Angelicae Sinensis *(Dang Gui)*
Semen Cuscutae Chinensis *(Tu Si Zi)*
Gelatinum Cornu Cervi *(Lu Jiao Jiao)*

Please note that the internal use of *Fu Zi* is currently not allowed in the UK. It is one of the most important herbs in Chinese medicine and we practitioners hope that this is a temporary situation. It should, however, never be taken without professional guidance.

Jin Gui Shen Qi Wan

Jin Gui is a reference to the name of the book this formula is taken from, *The Golden Cabinet*, a book written in approximately 250 AD. The rest of the name means Kidney Qi Pills. Along with the preceding formula, this is one of the most well known formulae for supplementing kidney yang in Chinese medicine. The same caveats and cautions apply to its use as to the previous one. Its ingredients consist of:

Cooked Radix Rehmanniae *(Shu Di)*
Radix Lateralis Praeparatus Aconiti Carmichaeli *(Fu Zi)*
Cortex Cinnamomi Cassiae *(Rou Gui)*
Fructus Corni Officinalis *(Shan Zhu Yu)*
Radix Dioscoreae Oppositae *(Shan Yao)*
Sclerotium Poriae Cocos *(Fu Ling)*
Rhizoma Alismatis *(Ze Xie)*
Cortex Radicis Moutan *(Dan Pi)*

Bu Zhong Yi Qi Wan

The name of this formula translates as Supplement the Centre and Boost the Qi Pills. It strongly supplements spleen vacuity. It is commonly used to treat central qi fall, i.e. prolapse of the stomach, uterus or rectum due to spleen qi vacuity. It is a very complex formula with a wide range of indications. It supplements the spleen but also courses the liver and rectifies the qi. It is one of the most commonly prescribed of all Chinese herbal formulae and these pills can be combined with a number of others when spleen qi vacuity plays a significant role in someone's condition. Its ingredients are:

Radix Astragali Membranacei *(Huang Qi)*
Radix Panacis Ginseng *(Ren Shen)*
Radix Glycyrrhizae *(Gan Cao)*
Rhizoma Atractylodis Macrocephalae *(Bai Zhu)*
Radix Angelicae Sinensis *(Dang Gui)*

Pericarpium Citri Reticulatae *(Chen Pi)*
Rhizoma Cimicifugae *(Sheng Ma)*
Radix Bupleuri *(Chai Hu)*
Rhizoma Atractylodis Macrocephalae *(Bai Zhu)*

Xue Fu Zhu Yu Wan

The name of these pills in English is Blood Mansion Dispels Stasis Pills. They are a commonly used basic formula for the treatment of blood stasis conditions. They can either be used as the main treatment for a predominantly blood stasis pattern, or can be combined with other Chinese patent medicines when blood stasis plays a contributory role. Blood stasis pain is fixed in one spot, is typically severe and is often described as sharp, piercing or stabbing. Chronic diseases are often complicated by blood stasis. The ingredients in this formula consist of:

Semen Pruni Persicae *(Tao Ren)*
Flos Carthami Tinctorii *(Hong Hua)*
Radix Angelicae Sinensis *(Dang Gui)*
Radix Ligustici Wallichii *(Chuan Xiong)*
Radix Rubrus Paeoniae Lactiflorae *(Chi Shao)*
Radix Bupleuri *(Chai Hu)*
Radix Platycodi Grandiflori *(Jie Geng)*
Fructus Citri Aurantii *(Zhi Ke)*
Uncooked Radix Rehmanniae *(Sheng Di)*
Radix Glycyrrhizae *(Gan Cao)*

Yan Hu Suo Wan

Called Corydalis Pills in English, this Chinese patent medicine consists of only two ingredients:

Rhizoma Corydalis Yanhusuo *(Yuan Hu Suo)*
Radix Angelicae Dahuricae *(Bai Zhi)*

The first ingredient moves the qi and quickens the blood. It is an all-purpose pain-reliever, but is especially effective for pain due to blood stasis. The second ingredient, Angelica, strongly moves the qi. It also tends to rise to the head and treats headache very effectively. These pills can be added to almost any other formula in order to treat the symptoms of a currently occurring, acute headache. They are not meant for long-term use. They do not treat the root of the problem, only the symptom or so-called branch, but they do treat the symptom of pain, if due to blood stasis, very effectively.

Bao Ji Wan (also spelt *Po Chai Wan*)

These pills are a frequently used Chinese patent medicine for food stagnation that is due to excessive eating and drinking. They consist of a number of ingredients whose action is to disperse food and abduct or lead away stagnation. We often give them out at parties when our guests may have eaten too much, and I have often taken one or two before bed when I have come home from a party or a restaurant where I may have eaten too much. The Chinese name translates as Protect (from) Accumulation Pills. Another similar pill is called *Kang Ning Wan*, Health Stabilising Pills. They are also sold under the name Curing Pills. The ingredients are a little different, but the action of these two formulae is very similar. Another such patent remedy for food stagnation is *Bao He Wan*, Protect Harmony Pills. The ingredients in this last formula are:

Massa Medica Fermentata *(Shen Qu)*
Fructus Crataegi *(Shan Zha)*
Semen Raphani Sativi *(Lai Fu Zi)*
Rhizoma Pinelliae Ternatae *(Ban Xia)*
Sclerotium Poriae Cocos *(Fu Ling)*
Pericarpium Citri Reticulatae *(Chen Pi)*
Fructus Forsythiae Suspensae *(Lian Qiao)*
Fructus Germinatus Hordei Vulgaris *(Mai Ya)*

These two formulae are probably the most well known and commonly used in the USA where they are currently available over the counter at American health food shops and at Asian speciality food shops.

I have tried to give you a selection of patent medicines that can be used to treat all the patterns of headache described earlier. There are many other important formulae and it may be that you require something different or more tailored to your individual needs. Should you choose to try Chinese herbal patent medicines for your headaches without supervision or guidance, please be careful. Be sure to follow the six guideposts below for assessing the safety of any medications you take.

ASSESSING OVER-THE-COUNTER MEDICATION

If you do try Chinese herbal patent medicines for your headache without professional guidance, please take great care to follow these guidelines for assessing the safety of any medications you take.

In general, you can tell if any medication and treatment is appropriate for you by checking the following six aspects of your health:

Digestion
Elimination
Energy level
Mood
Appetite
Sleep

If a medication, be it modern Western or traditional Chinese, alleviates your symptoms and these six basic areas of human health also improve, then it is probably a good treatment.

However, if a treatment or medication causes a deterioration in any of these six mechanisms, even if there is an improvement in your symptoms, then it is probably not the correct treatment and certainly should not be taken on a long-term basis. Chinese medicine aims to rebalance the body's energies and create harmony allowing the body's own natural healing mechanisms to be reinstated. Nothing is more powerful than nature's own healing and this is healing without side-effects.

ACUPUNCTURE AND ORIENTAL MEDICAL MASSAGE

I n the previous chapters we have looked at the underlying causes of headache from a traditional Chinese medicine (TCM) point of view, and its treatment with internal or herbal medicine. This chapter will focus on how Chinese medicine treats headache, using acupuncture and Oriental medical massage. Chinese medicine as it has evolved in China has developed in a different social and cultural context from the West and there are differences in how it is practised. In modern China, herbal treatment is very popular. In fact, TCM has evolved principally from a herbal tradition. In the West, there have been many other influences, and whilst TCM has played an important role, other countries, such as Japan, have also been influential. Shiatsu, for example, a type of Oriental medical massage originating from Japan, is very popular in the West today and can be a very helpful therapy for stress or tension headaches. Acupuncture is probably the most well known and widely practised form of Chinese medicine in the UK, having been practised since the 1960s. It has grown enormously in popularity and there are now many trained practitioners all over the UK. We will look at how to find a properly qualified practitioner later on in this book.

WHAT IS ACUPUNCTURE?

Acupuncture involves the insertion of extremely fine needles into specific points on the body along channels or pathways that correspond to the yin viscera and yang bowels we mentioned earlier. By stimulating these points, an acupuncturist may influence the flow of qi, or energy, in the pathway, thereby influencing the function of the corresponding viscus or bowel. Since all the viscera and bowels work together as a team, this then influences the whole energetic system of the person. The aim of acupuncture is to regulate the flow of qi so that there is more balance and harmony in the pathways or channels. Acupuncture can be very beneficial to treat headaches because it improves the flow of qi. The insertion of acupuncture needles at various points in the body moves the qi, which then moves the blood and body fluids. As soon as the flow of qi, blood and body fluids is normalised, the headache disappears. It is the lack of free flow that causes the pain. As the effect of acupuncture is immediate, it is an especially good first-aid remedy for a headache. Acupuncture may help to rectify and balance the flow of qi in the body and thereby improve overall health as well as relieving or improving specific or acute symptoms.

Acupuncture includes several other methods apart from the use of needles of stimulating acupuncture points to regulate the flow of qi in the body. One of these is moxibustion (see page 117). This means the warming of acupuncture points mainly by burning dried, aged, Oriental mugwort on, near or over acupuncture points. The purpose of this warming treatment is to stimulate the flow of qi and blood even more strongly, to add warmth to areas of the body that are too cold and to add yang qi to the body to supplement a yang qi deficiency. Some other methods or techniques to stimulate the points that may be used by the acupuncturist are cupping, electro-acupuncture and the application of magnets.

ACUPUNCTURE TREATMENT FOR HEADACHE

There are quite a few styles of acupuncture so some aspects of treatment will vary from practitioner to practitioner, depending on their training, but there are also certain aspects that remain the same. All practitioners will take a case history and gather together information so that they can make a diagnosis. They will almost certainly take the pulse at the wrist, examine the tongue and palpate the abdomen and the 'channels', looking for areas of tenderness or pain. Once a diagnosis has been made, the practitioner will select points along the channels and will stimulate these points using needles, moxa and possibly some of the other stimulation methods mentioned on page 82. These days most acupuncturists use disposable needles and all members of the professional bodies listed in this book must comply with strict standards of hygiene and safety. An acupuncture needle is extremely fine, nothing like a hypodermic needle, and although pain thresholds vary from person to person it is not necessarily a painful therapy. The effect of the treatment may be quite relaxing or even stimulating, as the qi is able to flow more freely in the body.

In China, acupuncture treatments are given every day or three to five times per week, depending on the nature and severity of the condition. In the West, however, health care delivery differs greatly from China, and it is not really feasible for patients to receive as many treatments per week. Western patients suffering from headaches usually respond well to acupuncture treatments performed once or twice a week for the first few weeks, followed by treatment once a week for a longer period. For chronic headaches, after an initial course of 10–12 sessions, it is best to continue acupuncture treatments once a month for a while. When the situation has improved, you can continue having treatment on a less frequent basis to maintain your health or return if you start having problems again.

In my clinical experience, if acupuncture is combined with appropriate diet and lifestyle changes, Chinese herbs and a selection of the self-care treatments recommended later

on in the book, the results will be even quicker and the relief
of symptoms even more complete.

How are the points selected?

The points the acupuncturist chooses to stimulate during
each treatment are selected on the basis of Chinese medical
theory and the known clinical effects of certain points. Since
there are different schools or styles of acupuncture, point
selection will vary from practitioner to practitioner. Here is
how a practitioner might treat a patient with a liver yang
hyperactivity pattern headache, based on Chinese medical
pattern discrimination.

Let's take the case of Jean, whom we saw before. She has
been able to come for a treatment during a migraine attack in
progress. Her main complaint is a severe, pounding pain in
the left side of her head. We previously established that Jean's
Chinese pattern discrimination is liver yang hyperactivity,
complicated by blood vacuity, which is, in turn, due to spleen
vacuity. During this acute episode, we are only going to
address the liver yang hyperactivity.

The treatment principles necessary for remedying this
case are to soothe the liver and reverse upward counterflow,
subdue yang and stop pain. In order to accomplish these
aims, the practitioner might select the following points:

Tai Chong (Liver 3)
He Gu (Large Intestine 4)
Wai Guan (Triple Burner 5)
Zu Lin Qi (Gall bladder 41)
Feng Chi (Gall bladder 20)
Tai Yang (extra channel point)
A shi (points of special pain)

The action of the points is as follows: *Tai Chong* courses the
liver and resolves depression, moves and rectifies the qi.

Rectification of the qi includes the reversing of upward counterflow.

He Gu is a widely used point with a variety of indications, depending on how it is used and with what points it is combined. *Hei Gu* and *Tai Chong* combined are known as 'the four gates'. They are used to free the flow in the entire body and to promote the upbearing of the clear and downbearing of the turbid by the qi mechanism. When used together, these points have a strong effect in relieving qi stagnation. In addition, *He Gu* is a very important point for the head and face.

Wai Guan and *Zu Lin Qi* form another frequently used two-point combination. *Wai Guan* is a point on the triple burner channel, while *Zu Lin Qi* is a point on the gall bladder channel. A headache on the side of the head means that the pain is due to a lack of free flow in these two channels which, together, make up the *shao yang*. Stimulating these two points on the affected side only helps to free the flow in the *shao yang*. This is a well known combination for treating headaches affecting the side of the head.

Feng Chi is also a *shao yang* gall bladder channel point. It is chosen for the same reason. It frees the flow of the *shao yang* in the affected area. It is combined with *Tai Yang*, one of the most important extra or non-channel points in the body. The name *Tai Yang* means supreme or greatest yang. Therefore, this point is particularly effective in treating hyperactive yang conditions resulting in symptoms manifesting in the head and is even more effective if those symptoms involve the side of the head.

A shi points include any point that, when pressed, elicits a pain response. In Jean's case, I would stimulate the places on the side of the head where she said the pain was particularly located. If Jean said that it hurt, then I would add between one and four *a shi* points to the standard points given above.

This combination of points addresses both Jean's Chinese pattern discrimination and her major complaint of pain. It remedies the underlying disease mechanism and addresses the key symptom of that mechanism in a very immediate way. It provides symptomatic relief at the same time as it corrects the underlying mechanisms of these symptoms.

Does acupuncture hurt?

The needles used in acupuncture are very fine and they are usually only inserted shallowly. It is not normally a painful experience although you may feel a slight soreness, heaviness or tingling where the needle is inserted. Japanese techniques using needles in particular are usually completely painless.

How quickly will I feel the result?

One of the best things about the acupuncture treatment of headache is that its effects are often immediate. Since many of the mechanisms of headache have to do with blocked qi, as soon as the qi is made to flow, the symptoms disappear. Many patients begin to feel better after the very first treatment.

Additionally, since irritability and nervous tension are mostly due to liver depression qi stagnation, people often will feel an immediate relief of irritability and tension while still on the treatment couch. Typically, you will feel a sense of pronounced tranquillity and relaxation within five to ten minutes of the insertion of the needles. Many patients do drop off to sleep for a few minutes while the needles are in place.

Who should receive acupuncture?

Since acupuncture often has an immediate effect on relieving a headache, it is a very good treatment. It is, however, particularly effective for liver yang hyperactivity, liver fire exuberance, phlegm dampness, food retention and blood stasis patterns of headache.

When a person's headaches are mostly due to qi vacuity, blood vacuity, yin or yang vacuity, then acupuncture is more effective when combined with Chinese herbal medicine. Although moxibustion can to a certain extent add yang qi to the body, acupuncture needles cannot add qi, blood or yin to a body in short supply of these. The most acupuncture can do in these cases is to stimulate the various viscera and bowels that engender and transform the qi, blood and yin. Chinese herbs, on the other hand, can directly introduce qi, blood and yin into the body, thus supplementing vacuities and deficiencies of these. If your headaches are due to a pronounced deficiency of qi, blood and/or yin, you should use acupuncture in combination with Chinese herbs.

Ear acupuncture

Some acupuncturists may also use points in the ear to treat headaches. Ear acupuncture is based on the idea that the ear looks like an upside-down foetus with the ear lobe representing the head. Points on the ear therefore correspond with areas of the body. Needles may be used to stimulate the points during the acupuncture session or alternatively tiny metal pellets, seeds or special 'press tac' needles are used, which are covered up with micropore or tape and left in place for a few days. In this way the effectiveness and duration of treatment may be enhanced.

In terms of headache, there are points in the ear that seem to correspond with, and affect, the head, as well as points that correspond to the liver, gall bladder, spleen, stomach and kidneys, all the viscera and bowels that participate in the various Chinese disease mechanisms of headache. Other points on the ear, such as Spirit Gate, Sympathetic Point, Brain Point and Subcortex Point, are very effective for relieving stress and generally calming the nervous system.

ORIENTAL MEDICAL MASSAGE

Medical massage in China is called *tui na*. It has developed into a high art and is practised extensively in hospitals and clinics. Like acupuncture, it works by stimulating the flow of qi in the channel or meridian system, except instead of needles, specific strokes or manipulations are used. At present there are not many trained *tui na* practitioners in the UK although it is growing in popularity. Another form of Oriental medical massage is shiatsu, which originates from Japan. This is a deeply relaxing therapy and there are a number of practitioners working in the UK. Shiatsu is done with the patient wearing loose comfortable clothing. Diagnosis is mainly through palpating the abdomen and channels to detect underlying imbalances in the person's energy. The relevant channels or meridians are then worked on to release blockages and strengthen areas of vacuity or deficiency. It may be very beneficial for headaches. Oriental medical massage can stimulate the flow of qi and it can also be very relaxing, making it an ideal treatment for sufferers of tension headaches. It is not even necessary to visit a therapist – self-massage techniques can be used for quick relief. For details, see pages 112–17.

THE THREE FREE THERAPIES

All the treatments and therapies we have discussed so far require the aid of a professional practitioner. There are however three 'free' therapies that are crucial to treating headaches. These are diet, exercise and deep relaxation. Only you can look after or take care of these three factors in your health!

DIET

As I have said earlier, in Chinese medicine, the function of the spleen and stomach are likened to a pot on a stove or a still. The stomach receives the foods and liquids, which are then processed into a mash. The spleen then cooks this mash and drives off (i.e. transforms and moves upwards) the pure part. This pure part collects in the lungs to become the qi and in the heart to become the blood. Chinese medicine characterises this transformation as a process of yang qi transforming yin substance. All the principles of Chinese dietary therapy that may be applied to treat and alleviate headaches are derived from these basic theories.

We have already seen that the spleen is the root of qi and blood engenderment and transformation. The spleen is also in charge of the movement and transformation of body fluids. Based on these facts, a healthy, strong spleen prevents and treats headaches in several ways. First of all, a strong spleen is one way of keeping the liver in check. It is said that once the liver is diseased, the next most likely viscus to be affected is the spleen. It is also said, 'When the liver is diseased, first treat the spleen.' Secondly, if the spleen is healthy and strong, it will create sufficient qi to push the blood and move body fluids. Having a sufficiency of pushing or moving spleen qi helps counterbalance or control any tendency to either blood stasis or phlegm dampness. Thirdly, the spleen is the root of blood production. A healthy spleen ensures there is sufficient blood to nourish and soften the liver, and to fill the brain. Additionally, excess blood not consumed by life's activities is converted into yin essence to be stored in the kidneys. Supplementing the spleen in order to nourish the blood is an indirect way of enriching and supplementing kidney yin. Excess qi is turned into yang essence, so supplementing the spleen in order to boost the qi is an indirect way of invigorating and supplementing kidney yang.

With regard to Chinese dietary therapy and headaches, the fundamental principle is to avoid foods that damage the spleen. These foods also typically produce dampness and phlegm.

Foods that damage the spleen

We begin with uncooked and, especially, chilled foods. In Chinese medicine, the process of cooking is seen as a type of predigestion before the food enters the body. It is therefore desirable that the overwhelming majority of all food to be eaten should be cooked, i.e. predigested. Although cooking may destroy some vital nutrients (in Chinese, qi), cooking does render the remaining nutrients into a more easily assimilated form. This means that even though some nutrients have been lost, the net absorption of nutrients is greater with cooked foods than raw. Furthermore, eating raw foods makes the spleen work harder and can overtax it. If one's spleen is very robust, eating uncooked, raw foods may not be too damaging, but women in particular need to take extra care as their monthly menses and resulting extra blood production may already be overtaxing the spleen. It is also a fact of life, according to Chinese medicine, that the spleen typically weakens with age.

Chilled foods even more than raw foods may directly damage the spleen. Chilled or frozen food and drink neutralise the spleen's yang qi. The process of digestion involves heating and digesting all food and drink to a warm soup within the stomach so that it may undergo 'distillation'. If the spleen expends too much yang qi just warming the food up, then it will become damaged and weak. So food and drink should be consumed at room temperature at the least and preferably at body temperature. The more signs and symptoms of spleen vacuity or deficiency that a person presents, such as fatigue, chronically loose stools, undigested food in the stools, cold hands and feet, dizziness on standing up and aversion to cold, the more they need to avoid uncooked, chilled food and drink.

Additionally, an excess of sugars and sweet things will directly damage the spleen. It is considered according to Chinese medicine that they are inherently dampening. This is because the body creates or secretes fluids that gather and transform into dampness in response to an excess of sweet food and drink. The spleen is averse to dampness. Dampness is a yin substance and controls or checks yang qi, which is very important to the proper functioning of the spleen. So anything that is excessively dampening damages the spleen. The sweeter a food is, the more dampening and, therefore, more damaging it is to the spleen.

Other food categories considered to be dampening and subsequently damaging to the spleen are:

'Sodden wheat' foods
This means flour products, such as bread and noodles. Wheat (as opposed to rice) is damp in its nature. When it is steamed, yeasted and/or refined, it becomes even more damp.

Oils and fats

The more oily or greasy a food is, the worse it is for the spleen. As milk contains a lot of fat, dairy products fall into this category. This includes milk, butter and cheese.

If we add all this up, then ice cream is just about the worst thing a person with a weak, damp spleen could eat. Ice cream is chilled, it is intensely sweet and it is filled with fat. So it is a triple whammy when it comes to damaging the spleen. Pasta smothered in tomato sauce and cheese is another recipe for disaster. Pasta made from wheat flour is dampening, tomatoes are dampening, and cheese is dampening. Fruit juice is also very damaging to the spleen and produces damp – a glass of fruit juice contains as much sugar as a bar of chocolate.

Below is a list of Western foods that are either uncooked, chilled, too sweet or too dampening and thus damaging to the spleen. People suffering from headaches due to or involving qi vacuity, blood vacuity, phlegm dampness or food stagnation should minimise or avoid these foods according to how weak and damp their spleen is.

Ice cream
Sugar
Sweets, especially chocolate
Milk
Butter
Cheese
Margarine
Yoghurt
Raw salads
Fruit juices
Juicy, sweet fruits, such as oranges, peaches, strawberries and
    tomatoes
Fatty meats

Fried foods
Refined flour products – cakes and biscuits
Yeasted bread
Nuts
Alcohol

If the spleen is weak and wet, it is best not to eat too much of anything at any one time. A weak spleen can be overwhelmed by a large meal, especially if any of the food is hard to digest. This then results in food stagnation, which impedes the free flow of qi all the more and causes further damage to the spleen.

A clear, bland diet

In Chinese medicine, the best diet for the spleen and, therefore, for most people, is what is called a 'clear, bland diet'. This is a diet high in complex carbohydrates such as unrefined grains, especially rice and beans. It contains a large proportion of lightly cooked vegetables. It is a diet that avoids fatty meats, oily, greasy, fried foods and very sweet foods. It is not, however, a completely vegetarian diet. Most people, in my experience, should eat one to two ounces of various types of meat two to four times per week. This animal flesh could be chicken and fish, but should also include some lean beef, pork and lamb. Some fresh or cooked fruits may be eaten, but fruit juices should be avoided. Women especially should make an effort to include tofu and tempeh, two soya foods now commonly available in health food shops and good supermarkets, in their diet.

If the spleen is weak, then it is best to eat smaller meals and eat more frequently. Rice is an excellent food for three reasons: firstly it is neutral in temperature, secondly it fortifies the spleen, thereby supplementing the qi, and thirdly it eliminates dampness. Rice should be the main grain in the diet.

A few problem foods

There are a few 'problem' foods that deserve special mention.

Coffee

Many people crave coffee for two reasons. Firstly, coffee moves blocked qi. So, if a person suffers from liver depression qi stagnation, coffee will temporarily make them feel as though their qi is flowing. Secondly, coffee transforms essence into qi and makes that qi temporarily available to the body. This means that people who suffer from spleen and/or kidney vacuity fatigue will get a temporary lift from coffee. It will make them feel as if they have energy. Once this energy is used up, however, they are left with a negative deficit. The coffee has transformed some of the essence stored in the kidneys into qi. This qi has been used, and now there is less stored essence. Since the blood and essence share a common source, coffee drinking may ultimately worsen headaches associated with blood or kidney vacuities. Tea has a similar effect in that it transforms yin essence into yang qi but the quantity of caffeine in black tea is usually only half that found in coffee.

Chocolate

Another problem food is chocolate. Chocolate is a combination of oil, sugar and cocoa. We have seen that both oil and sugar are dampening and damaging to the spleen. Temporarily, the sugar will boost the spleen qi, but ultimately it will result in 'sugar blues' or a hypoglycaemic let-down. Cocoa stirs the life gate fire. The life gate fire is another name for kidney yang or kidney fire, and kidney fire is the source of sexual energy and desire. It is said that chocolate is the food of love and, from the Chinese medical point of view, that is true. Since chocolate stimulates kidney fire at the same time as it temporarily boosts the spleen, it does produce a rush of yang qi. This rush of yang qi moves depression and stagnation, at least in the short term. So it makes sense that some people with liver depression, spleen vacuity and kidney yang debility might crave chocolate.

Alcohol

Alcohol is damp and hot, according to Chinese medical theory. It strongly moves the qi and blood. So people with liver depression qi stagnation will feel temporarily better after drinking alcohol. However, the sugar in alcohol damages the spleen and creates dampness that 'gums up the works' whilst the heat (yang) in alcohol can waste the blood (yin) and aggravate depressive liver heat and/or hyperactive liver yang.

Hot, peppery foods

Spicy, peppery, 'hot' foods also move the qi, thereby temporarily relieving liver depression qi stagnation. However, like alcohol, the heat in spicy hot foods wastes the blood and can inflame yang.

Sour foods

In Chinese medicine, the sour flavour is inherently astringent and constricting. People with liver depression qi stagnation should be careful not to use vinegar and other intensely sour foods. Such sour flavoured foods will only aggravate the qi stagnation by further restricting the qi and blood. This is also why sweet and sour foods, such as orange juice and tomatoes, are particularly bad for people with liver depression and spleen vacuity. The sour flavour constricts the qi, while the sweet flavour damages the spleen and creates dampness.

Foods that help nourish the blood
Qi and wei

According to Chinese dietary therapy, all foods contain both qi and wei in varying amounts. Qi means the ability to catalyse or promote yang function, while wei (literally translated as flavour) refers to a food's ability to nourish or construct yin substance. Since blood is relatively yin compared to qi being yang, a certain amount of food high in wei is necessary for a person to create and transform blood. Foods that are high in wei as compared to qi tend to be heavy, dense, greasy or oily, meaty or bloody. All animal products contain more wei than vegetable products. Black beans or, even better, black soya beans contain more wei than celery or lettuce.

When people suffer from headaches due to blood vacuity failing to nourish the brain, they usually need to eat slightly more foods high in wei. This includes animal proteins and products, such as meat and eggs. According to Chinese medicine flesh foods are very 'compassionate' to the human body. This word recognises the fact that the animal's life has had to be sacrificed to produce this type of food. It also recognises that, because such food is so close to the human body itself, it is especially nutritious. Eating some animal products can therefore be helpful and may even be necessary when people suffer from headaches with blood vacuity.

Animal foods versus vegetarianism

In my many years of clinical experience, I have observed that many Westerners who adhere to a strict vegetarian diet develop blood or yin vacuity patterns after several years. This is especially the case in women who lose blood every month and must build babies out of the blood and yin essence. When women who are strict vegetarians come to see me, if they present the signs and symptoms of blood vacuity (a thick, pale tongue, pale face, nails and lips, heart palpitations, insomnia and fatigue with a fine, forceless pulse), I recommend that they include a little animal food in their diet. They often report to me how much better they feel once they have made these dietary changes.

The downside of eating meat, apart from ethical issues, is that foods that are high in wei also tend to be harder to digest and to create phlegm and dampness. It is best that such foods should only be eaten in very small amounts at any one time. The weaker the person's spleen or the more phlegm and dampness they already have, the less of such foods they should eat.

Remember that the process of digestion first consisted of turning the food and drink ingested into a warm soup in the stomach. Soups and broths made out of animal flesh are the easiest and most digestible way of adding some animal-quality wei to the diet. Flesh itself should probably be limited to only one to two ounces (25–50 grams) per serving and only three or four such servings per week. According to Chinese dietary principles, the best meats for creating and transforming blood and yin essence are offal and red or dark meats. This includes beef, venison and lamb and dark meat from chicken, turkey, goose and duck. White pork meat and ham are also good but white fish and white poultry meat are less effective for building blood.

One good recipe for adding more digestible wei to the diet of a person who is blood vacuous is to boil a marrow bone with some cut vegetables, especially root vegetables, and black beans or black soya beans. The resulting soup is easy to digest and yet rich in wei.

In the following chapter, the reader will find some specific recipes combining Chinese herbs and foods to treat or prevent various patterns of headache.

Some last words on diet

In conclusion, Western patients are always asking me what they should eat in order to get rid of their headaches. When it comes to diet, however, sad to say, the issue is not so much what to eat as what not to eat. Diet most definitely plays a major role in the cause and perpetuation of many headaches, but, except in the case of vegetarians suffering from blood or yin vacuities, the issue is mainly what to avoid or minimise, not what to add. Most of us know that coffee, chocolate, sugars and sweets, oils and fats and alcohol are not good for us. Most of us know that we should be eating more complex carbohydrates and freshly cooked vegetables and less fatty meat. However, it's one thing to know these things and another to follow what we know.

To be perfectly honest, a clear, bland diet as recommended according to the principles of Chinese medicine is not the most exciting diet in the world. It is, however, quite a traditional type of diet and many of our great-grandparents would have eaten like this. Our modern Western diet, which is high in oils and fats, high in sugars and sweets, high in animal proteins and proportionally high in uncooked, chilled foods and drinks, is a relatively recent phenomenon, and you can't fool Mother Nature.

When you change to the clear, bland diet of Chinese medicine, you may find that at first you suffer from cravings for more tasty food. These cravings are, in many cases, actually associated with food 'allergies'. We crave what is actually not good for us in the same way that an alcoholic craves for alcohol. After a few days, however, these cravings tend to disappear and you can find that you don't miss some of the convenience or 'comfort' foods as much as you thought you would. Perseverance is the key to long-term success. As the Chinese say, 'A million is made up of nothing but lots of ones, and a bucket is quickly filled by steady drips and drops.'

EXERCISE

Exercise is the second of the three free therapies. According to Chinese medicine, regular and adequate exercise has two basic benefits. Firstly, exercise promotes the movement of the qi and quickening of the blood. Since all headaches involve a lack of free flow, it is obvious that exercise is an important therapy for moving the qi and quickening the blood. Secondly, exercise benefits the spleen. The spleen's movement and transportation of digested food is dependent upon the qi mechanism. The qi mechanism describes the function of the qi in moving up and down the clear and turbid parts of digestion respectively. For the qi mechanism to function properly, the qi must be flowing normally and freely. Since exercise moves and rectifies the qi, it also helps regulate and rectify the qi mechanism. The result is that the spleen is able to function well, creating and transforming qi and blood. Spleen qi vacuity and dampness accumulation typically complicate many people's headaches; a healthy spleen is able to check or keep under control a depressed or hyperactive liver. Regular, adequate exercise can be a vitally important component for any person who suffers from headaches on a regular basis.

Aerobics

In my experience, I find aerobic exercise to be the most beneficial for the majority of people with headaches. By aerobic exercise, I mean any physical activity that raises the heartbeat 80 per cent above normal resting rate and keeps it there for at least 20 minutes. To calculate your normal resting heart rate, place your fingers over the pulsing artery on the front side of your neck. Count the beats for 15 seconds and then multiply by four. This gives you your beats per minute or BPM. Now multiply your BPM by 0.8. Take the resulting number and add it to your resting BPM. This gives you your aerobic threshold of BPM. Next engage in any physical activity you like. After you have been exercising for five minutes, take your pulse for 15 seconds once again at the artery on the front side of your throat. Again multiply the resulting count by four and this tells you your current BPM. If this number is less than your aerobic threshold BPM, then you know you need to exercise harder or faster. Once you get your heart rate up to your aerobic threshold, then you need to keep exercising at the same level of intensity for at least 20 minutes. Take your pulse every five minutes or so to ensure your heartbeat is being kept high enough.

Depending on your age and physical condition, you will require different types of exercise to reach your aerobic threshold. For some people, simply walking briskly will raise their heartbeat 80 per cent above its resting rate. Others will need to do calisthenics, running, swimming, squash or some other more strenuous exercise. It really does not matter what the exercise is as long as it raises your heartbeat 80 per cent above your resting rate and keeps it there for 20 minutes. My advice is that you go for something you enjoy and don't find too boring, otherwise you won't want to keep it up. You should also try to make sure that it doesn't cause you any problems or damage to any parts of the body. For example, running on pavements may damage the knees.

When doing aerobic exercise, it is best to exercise either every day or every other day. If you do not do your aerobics at least once every 72 hours, then its cumulative effects won't be as good. I recommend that my patients with headaches do some sort of aerobic exercises every day or every other day, three to four times per week at least. The good news is that there is no real need to exercise more than 30 minutes at any one time. A session of 45 minutes is not going to be all that much better than 25 minutes, and 25 minutes four times per week is very much better than one hour once a week.

Too much exercise

Whilst the vast majority of people suffering from headaches will benefit from doing more exercise, there are a few for whom it could be harmful. According to Chinese medical theory, all activity entails a consumption of yin by yang. If someone is constitutionally deficient in yin due to circumstances such as ageing, persistent illness, extreme blood loss, excessive births or lactation, then too much exercise or physical activity can worsen the situation. This condition can be seen in women with thin bodily constitutions who over-exercise, such as professional athletes, or in women who suffer from anorexia or bulimia.

Body fat in Chinese medicine is considered to be yin, so someone who is very thinly built tends to have less yin to start off with. If the body fat is further reduced through exercise, it may become so insufficient that yin can no longer control yang. In women, such a deficiency of yin blood because of too much exercise usually manifests first in the cessation of menstruation (amenorrhoea). It is also possible for use of drugs, especially amphetamines or 'speed', and eating disorders such as anorexia and bulimia to result in an over-consumption of yin. This can lead to amenorrhoea, increased mental agitation and insomnia. In the case of bulimia, although the person is eating, they are not getting sufficient yin nourishment as they are bingeing and purging.

You will know that the amount of exercise you do is correct if you feel refreshed and invigorated a couple of hours after the exercise is over. If you notice that you feel even more fatigued or nervous and jittery, or if exercise during the day leads to night sweats and insomnia, then you need to reduce your level of exercise.

DEEP RELAXATION

As we have seen, headaches are frequently associated with hyperactive liver yang counterflowing upwards, and hyperactive liver yang typically evolves from long-term or severe liver depression qi stagnation. If liver depression is long-lasting or severe, it can transform into heat or fire, which, being yang, consume and exhaust yin and blood. Yang qi then moves frenetically upwards to crash into the 'bony box' of the skull. Therefore, liver depression qi stagnation is often at the root of headache. In Chinese medicine, liver depression comes from stress, frustration and emotional upset, which is why to a certain extent it is endemic amongst adults living in today's hectic world. Also in Chinese medicine, anger relates to the venting of pent-up qi in the liver. When qi becomes depressed in the liver, it accumulates like hot air in a balloon so when there is a little more frustration or stress, it vents itself upwards and is expressed as irritability, anger or shouting, or as headache, dizziness, vertigo and facial nervous tics. In Chinese medicine, it is a statement of fact that 'Anger results in the qi ascending.'

Essentially, this type of anger is due to a maladoptive coping response, probably learned at a young age. When we feel frustrated or stressed by something, most of us tense our muscles, particularly those in our upper back and shoulders, neck and jaws. We also probably hold our breath. In Chinese medicine, the sinews are governed by the liver. This tensing of the muscles, or the sinews, constricts the flow of qi in the channels and network vessels, and because the liver is responsible for the coursing and discharging of this qi, such tensing of the sinews leads to liver depression qi stagnation. Since the lungs govern the downward spreading and movement of the qi, holding our breath due to stress or frustration only worsens this tendency of the qi not to move and to become depressed and stagnant.

So, deep relaxation is the third of the free therapies. For deep relaxation to be therapeutic medically, it needs to be more than just mental equilibrium. It needs to be physical or bodily relaxation as well as mental repose. Most of us are not able to sense that every thought we think and feeling we feel actually corresponds to a physical sensation somewhere in our body. The words we use to describe emotions are all abstract nouns, such as anger, depression, sadness and melancholy. In Chinese medicine, every emotion is associated with a change in the direction or flow of qi. Anger makes the qi move upwards. Fear, on the other hand, makes the qi move downwards. Anger 'makes our gorge rise' or 'blows our top', while fear may cause a 'sinking feeling'. These colloquial expressions are all based on the age-old wisdom that all thoughts and emotions are not just mental but also bodily events. This is why it is not just enough to clear your mind. Clearing your mind is good, but for really marked therapeutic results, it is even better if you clear your mind whilst relaxing every muscle in your body as well as your breathing.

Relaxation tapes

An effective way to practise such mental and physical deep relaxation is to listen to a daily, guided, deep relaxation audiotape. It is guided in the sense that a narrator on the tape leads you through the process of deep relaxation. These tapes normally lead you to relax the body in a progressive manner, first relaxing one part and then moving on to another.

There are many such tapes available, usually sold in health food shops or good bookshops. Choose several tapes so that you won't get too bored of listening to the same one. When looking for a good relaxation tape, firstly ensure that the tape is a guided tape and not a subliminal relaxation tape. Subliminal tapes usually have music and any instructions to relax are given so quietly that they are not consciously heard.

Although such tapes can help you feel relaxed when you use them, ultimately they do not teach you how to relax as a skill that you can then consciously practise. Secondly, make sure the tape starts from the top of the body and works downwards. This is because anger makes the qi go upwards in the body; frustration and anger due to liver depression qi stagnation mean there is already too much qi rising upwards in the body. This depressed qi needs not only to be moved but to be moved downwards. Thirdly, make sure the tape instructs you to relax your physical body. If you do not relax all your muscles or sinews, the qi cannot flow freely and the liver cannot be coursed. The tape will not be as beneficial if you don't relax your muscles. Finally, try to make sure the tape instructs you to let your breath go with each exhalation. One of the symptoms of liver depression is a stuffy feeling in the chest that we unconsciously try to relieve by sighing. Letting each exhalation go completely helps the lungs push the qi downwards.

The importance of daily practice

I was once taken on a field trip to a hospital clinic in Shanghai where they were using deep relaxation as a therapy with patients suffering from high blood pressure, heart disease, strokes, migraines and insomnia. The doctors at this clinic showed us various graphs plotting their research data on how such daily, progressive deep relaxation can regulate the blood pressure and body temperature and improve the appetite, digestion, elimination, sleep, energy and mood. One of the things they said has stuck with me for 15 years: 'Small results in 100 days, big results in 1,000.' This means that if one does such daily, progressive deep relaxation every single day for 100 days, one will definitely experience certain results. What are these 'small' results? They are improvements in all the parameters listed before: blood pressure, body temperature, appetite, digestion, elimination, sleep, energy and mood. The 'big' results experienced after 1,000 days of practice are a change in how one reacts to stress – in other words, a change in one's very personality or character.

What these doctors in Shanghai stressed and what I have also experienced both personally and with my patients is that the effects of this relaxation are cumulative. This means that the longer one can practise this routine on a consistent daily basis, the greater and more lasting the effects will be.

It is vitally important to do such daily, guided, progressive, deep relaxation every single day, day in and day out for a solid three months at least and for a continuous three years at best. If one does such progressive, somatic, deep relaxation every day, one will see every parameter or measurement of health and well-being improve. If one does this kind of deep relaxation only sporadically, missing a day here and there, it will feel good when you do it, but it will not have the marked, cumulative therapeutic effects it can. Perseverance is the real key to getting the benefits of deep relaxation.

The real test

Doing such a daily deep relaxation regime is only practice, however. It's like hitting tennis balls against a wall or hitting a bucket of balls at a driving range: it is not the real game itself. The real purpose of a daily deep relaxation regime is not just to relieve immediate stress and strain, but to learn a new skill, a new way to react to stress. The ultimate goal is to learn how to breathe out and immediately relax all the muscles in the body in reaction to stress, rather than holding the breath and tensing up. By doing such deep relaxation day after day, one learns how to relax any and every muscle in the body quickly and efficiently. Then, as soon as you recognise that you are feeling frustrated, stressed out or uptight, you can immediately remedy those feelings at the same time as coursing your liver and rectifying your qi. This is the real test, the game of life. Remember: 'Small results in 100 days, big results in 1,000.'

SIMPLE HOME REMEDIES FOR HEADACHES

By changing your diet, getting adequate exercise and altering how you deal with stress in a fundamental way, you will significantly improve your health and have fewer headaches. These lifestyle changes are probably the most important things that you can do for yourself. In this chapter we will look at some simple home remedies based on Chinese medicine, which you may find useful to help relieve the symptoms of headache.

CHINESE AROMATHERAPY

In Chinese medicine, the qi is seen as a type of wind or vapour. The Chinese character for qi shows wind blowing over a rice field and an object's smell is often referred to as its qi. So, there is a close relationship between smells carried through the air and the flow of qi in a person's body. Although aromatherapy has been a major part of professionally practised Chinese medicine for almost 1,000 years, there is a simple aromatherapy treatment that one can do at home that can help alleviate irritability, depression, nervousness, anxiety and insomnia.

A ingredient often used in Asian incense is Lignum Aquilariae Agallochae (eaglewood). The Chinese name for it is *Chen Xiang*, which means 'sinking fragrance'. In Chinese medicine, Aquilaria is classified as a qi-rectifying medicinal. When used as a boiled decoction, or 'tea', Aquilaria moves the qi, stops pain and promotes the movement of the qi in a downward direction in the body. It is my belief that the reason it is called sinking fragrance has to do with this ability to move the qi downwards. When it is burnt as a medicinal incense it is very calming and soothing. You should be able to buy this herb from specialist Chinese herbal suppliers or shops. The powdered variety is best but if this is not available then you can powder your own in a coffee grinder or just use small pieces of the herb. You will also need to buy some incense charcoal. To carry out the treatment, light an incense charcoal in a flameproof dish and put a few small pinches of the Aquilaria on it. As the smoke rises, inhale deeply. This treatment can be carried out as needed or, if you are suffering from stress, repeat it at least three times a week. It will help with restlessness, nervousness, anxiety and irritability.

This Chinese aromatherapy with Lignum Aquilariae Agallochae is very effective. I know of no side-effects or contraindications.

INHALATION THERAPY

Somewhat similar to aromatherapy is inhalation therapy. The aromatherapy regime described above is meant primarily to treat liver depression qi stagnation, a condition which we have seen can lead to a headache. It does not, however, treat headaches *per se*. The following inhalation therapy is a first-aid treatment for headaches, meant actually to relieve the symptoms of pain in the head while they are occurring. Before you can use it, you will need to prepare the medicinal powder that you are going to inhale, which is made up of the following Chinese medicinals. Weigh each ingredient, then grind separately into a fine powder, before mixing them all together.

5 ml/1 tsp Radix Ligustici Wallichii *(Chuan Xiong)*
2.5 ml/½ tsp Herba Asari Cum Radice *(Xi Xin)*
5 ml/1 tsp Radix Et Rhizoma Notopterygii *(Qiang Huo)*
5 ml/1 tsp Flos Camelliae Sinensis *(Cha Ye)*
5 ml/1 tsp Herba Seu Flos Schizonepetae Tenuifoliae *(Jing Jie Sui)*

5 ml/1 tsp   Radix Platycodi Grandiflori *(Jie Geng)*
5 ml/1 tsp   Radix Ledebouriellae Divaricatae *(Fang Feng)*
5 ml/1 tsp   Radix Angelicae Dahuricae *(Bai Zhi)*
5 ml/1 tsp   Herba Menthae Haplocalycis *(Bo He)*

At the time of pain, inhale one tenth of one gram of this powder through the nostril on the affected side and then exhale through the mouth. If both sides are affected, then inhale one tenth of one gram through each nostril. One can repeat this at intervals of 15 minutes or more. Stop this therapy if it causes any breathing difficulty or pain or bleeding from the nose or sinus cavities. In most cases, this inhalant powder actually helps treat sinus infections. Details of where to obtain the herbs are given on pages 154–58.

CHINESE HERBAL PILLOW

The following recipe is for a Chinese herbal pillow. It can be used for those suffering from headaches of various patterns but is especially beneficial for those associated with blood stasis. The ingredients in this formula quicken the blood and dispel stasis. Weigh and grind the following medicinals into powder separately as before and sew them into a small, flat cotton bag just big enough to lay the head upon.

30 ml/2 tbsp   Radix Angelicae Sinensis *(Dang Gui)*
15 ml/1 tbsp   Radix Et Rhizoma Notopterygii *(Qiang Huo)*
30 ml/2 tbsp   Radix Ligustici Wallichii *(Chuan Xiong)*
7.5 ml/1½ tsp   Radix Lateralis Praeparatus Aconiti
                Carmichaeli *(Fu Zi)*
7.5 ml/1½ tsp   Radix Aconiti *(Chuan Wu)*
15 ml/1 tbsp   Radix Et Rhizoma Ligustici Chinensis *(Gao Ben)*
15 ml/1 tbsp   Radix Rubrus Paeoniae Lactiflorae *(Chi Shao)*
15 ml/1 tbsp   Flos Carthami Tinctorii *(Hong Hua)*
15 ml/1 tbsp   Lumbricus *(Di Long)*

15 ml/1 tbsp   Sanguis Draconis *(Xue Jie)*
15 ml/1 tbsp   Rhizoma Acori Graminei *(Shi Chang Pu)*
15 ml/1 tbsp   Medulla Junci *(Deng Xin Cao)*
7.5 ml/1½ tsp Herba Asari Cum Radice *(Xi Xin)*
15 ml/1 tbsp   Ramulus Cinnamomi Cassiae *(Gui Zhi)*
15 ml/1 tbsp   Radix Salviae Miltiorrhizae *(Dan Shen)*
15 ml/1 tbsp   Radix Ledebouriellae Divaricatae *(Fang Feng)*
15 ml/1 tbsp   Semen Raphani Sativi *(Lai Fu Zi)*
15 ml/1 tbsp   Radix Clematidis Chinensis *(Wei Ling Xian)*
15 ml/1 tbsp   Resina Olibani *(Ru Xiang)*
15 ml/1 tbsp   Resina Myrrhae *(Mo Yao)*
2 ml/½ tsp   Borneolum *(Bing Pian)*

One can then sleep on this pillow every night, placing that part of the head where the pain is the worst on top of the pillow. This formula is for external use only. It is not meant for internal administration. See page 154 for suppliers of Chinese herbs.

POULTICES AND PLASTERS

Below are a selection of Chinese herbal poultices and plasters for the treatment of various types of headaches. They are reasonably easy to make, relatively safe and quite effective. If any of them causes skin irritation or blistering, discontinue use immediately.

For liver yang headaches, take some Fructus Evodiae Rutecarpae *(Wu Zhu Yu)* and grind it into powder. Then mix some of this powder with a little vinegar. Make into a paste and apply to *Yong Quan* (Kidney 1) on the soles of the feet. Fix in place with sticking plaster and leave in place for one day. Do this once each day for seven days. If this causes a blister, take off the plaster and dress it as you would any blister.

Even though you have removed the plaster, its effect will continue. This simple plaster works by leading yang back down out of the head to its lower source in the kidneys.

For the first-aid treatment of various types of headache, mash 20 g of white onion. Then grind 20 g of Sichuan peppercorns and 12 g of Radix Ligustici Wallichii *(Chuan Xiong)*. Mix these together with a little peppermint oil and white flour and shape into flat herbal discs. Apply these discs to *Tai Yang* (the extra channel point) and *Bai Hui* (Governing Vessel 20). Hold in place with sticking plaster or tie in place with cotton gauze. Do this as needed.

For wind heat headache, take 15 g of Excrementum Bombycis *(Can Sha)* and 30 g of uncooked Gypsum Fibrosum *(Shi Gao)*. Grind these into fine powder and mix with a little vinegar into a paste. Apply this paste to the forehead once per day. Three to five applications equals one course of therapy.

For the first-aid relief of headache, take 12 g of Radix Angelicae Sinensis *(Dang Gui)*, 6 g of Radix Ligustici Wallichii *(Chuan Xiong)* and 6 g of Rhizoma Cyperi Rotundi *(Xiang Fu)*. Grind these into powder and mix with 20 g of table salt. Place this powder in a dry wok or pan and stir-fry till hot. Then wrap in clean cotton cloth and apply to the affected area of the head.

For headaches that are characterised by particularly severe wind cold, grind into powder 45 g each of Radix Et Rhizoma Notopterygii *(Qiang Huo)* and Radix Angelicae Pubescentis *(Du Huo)*, 30 g of Radix Rubrus Paeoniae Lactiflorae *(Chi Shao)*, 20 g of Radix Angelicae Dahuricae *(Bai Zhi)* and 18 g of

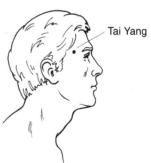
Tai Yang

Rhizoma Acori Graminei *(Shi Chang Pu)*. Then mix this with the juice pressed from five or more spring onions. Make this into a paste and then apply this paste to *Tai Yang, Feng Chi* (Gall Bladder 20), and *Feng Fu* (Governing Vessel 16).

Hold in place with a sticking plaster. Change once each day.

One more external remedy for a wind cold pattern headache is to take equal amounts of black pepper and Folium Artemisiae Argyii *(Ai Ye)*. Grind these into powder and then mix with a suitable amount of egg white. Apply this paste to Bai Hui (Governing Vessel 20) and change this once each day. Five to seven days equals one course of therapy.

CHINESE SELF-MASSAGE

Massage, including self-massage, is a highly developed part of traditional Chinese medicine. The self-massage regime which I have included here is specifically designed as a home remedy for headache. More Chinese self-massage regimes are described in Fan Ya-li's *Chinese Self-massage Therapy: The Easy Way to Health* (see page 168).

1. Press and knead the area between the eyebrows above the bridge of the nose. This is the acupuncture point *Yin Tang* and it is especially useful for calming the spirit and soothing the liver. Do this approximately 100 times.

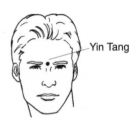

Yin Tang

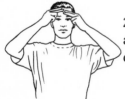

2. Rub the eyebrows with the thumbs and forefingers outwards from the centre. Do this 100 times.

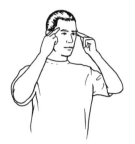

3. Rub the temples with the tips of the thumbs or middle fingers 100 times until there is a feeling of mild soreness and distention.

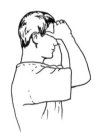

4. Rub the temples backwards with the edges of the thumbs 100 times, from the orbits of the eyes to within the hairline. Rub in only one direction – from front to back.

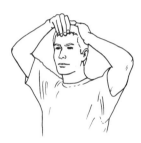

5. Place the fingers of one hand on the forehead so that the middle finger is in the middle of the forehead and the other fingers are just below the hairline to either side. The palm of the hand will be resting gently on the top of the head. Now massage backwards from the forehead to the centre of the top of the head 20–30 times, by tightening and relaxing the fingers.

6. Pat the top of the head with the hollow of the palm 30–50 times. The point in the middle of the top of the head is called *Bai Hui* (Meeting of Hundreds, Governing Vessel 20). Stimulation of this point calms the spirit and moves down upwardly counterflowing and exuberant liver yang.

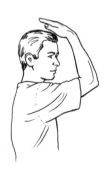

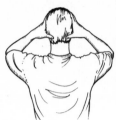

7. Press and knead the base of the skull in the depressions on both sides of the back of the neck. This is acupuncture point *Feng Chi* (Gall Bladder 20) and is a major point for relieving headaches arising from upwardly counterflowing liver qi. Do this approximately 100 times.

8. Pound the centre of the top of one shoulder with the opposite fist, loosely clenched. This is acupuncture point *Jian Jing* (Gall Bladder 21). It also moves down upwardly counterflowing liver qi. Do this 30–50 times on each side.

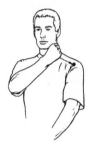

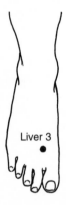

Liver 3

This self-massage regime is appropriate for premenstrual migraines and other types of headaches due to the upward counterflow of liver yang or liver fire. It should take 20–30 minutes. It can be done as a first-aid treatment for a headache currently underway. For severe, recurrent headaches, you can do this regime once a day or once every other day. In this case, finish by rubbing the thumbs alternately downwards over the point *Tai Chong* (Liver 3) located in the space between the first and second bones on the top of each foot (the metatarsals). Massaging this point like this drains the liver and downbears the qi. Do this 30–50 times.

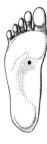

Then knead the point _Yong Quan_ (Kidney 1) in the hollow of the sole of the foot, just behind and to one side of the ball of the foot. Do this for 2–3 minutes per foot. This point enriches kidney yin and reverses upward counterflow, using kidney yin to control hyperactive liver yang.

SEVEN STAR HAMMERING

A seven star hammer is a small hammer or mallet with seven small needles embedded in its head. It is one of the ways of stimulating various acupuncture points without actually inserting a needle into the body. Seven star hammers can be useful to treat people who are frightened of needles, for children, or for those who wish to treat their own condition at home. When the points to be stimulated are on the front of the body, you can perform this technique on yourself. If they are located on the back of the body, this technique can be done by a family member or a friend. This is a very easy technique, which does not require any special training or expertise. Seven star hammers (also called plum blossom hammers and dermal needles) can be purchased from some of the suppliers listed on pages 154–58.

For headache due to invasion of external evils, such as wind cold or wind heat:

1. Tap the back of the neck, the upper back, and the region of the head affected by the pain. In particular, tap _Feng Chi_ (Gall Bladder 20).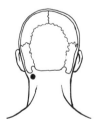

2. Tap *Tai Yang*.

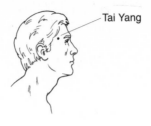

Tai Yang

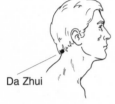

3. Tap *Da Zhui* (Governing Vessel 14).

Da Zhui

Tap *Tai Yang* and *Da Zhui* hard enough to make them bleed just a little. Clean the area with a sterile cotton ball dipped in alcohol or hydrogen peroxide.

For headache due to internal causes, including liver yang hyperactivity:
1. Tap the back of the neck and the affected area.
2. Tap *Tai Yang* (see above).

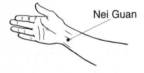

Nei Guan

3. Tap *Nei Guan* (Pericardium 6).

Wai Guan

4. Tap *Wai Guan* (Triple Burner 5).

Then tap the entire sacrum. Do all the above with moderate stimulation. If there is liver fire, tap *Tai Yang* hard enough so that it bleeds just a little. Then clean with cotton and alcohol or hydrogen peroxide as above. In general, any part of the head can be tapped with the seven star hammer where there is pain.

Between treatments, soak the seven star hammer in alcohol or hydrogen peroxide. To prevent any cross-infection do not share anyone else's hammer. Seven star hammers are very inexpensive, so each person can easily afford to have their own. For suppliers' names and addresses, see pages 154–58.

THREAD MOXIBUSTION

Thread moxibustion involves burning extremely tiny cones or 'threads' of aged Oriental mugwort directly on top of certain chosen points. When done correctly, this is a very simple and effective way of adding yang qi to the body without causing a burn or scar. This method is appropriate primarily for those who suffer from kidney yang vacuity headaches. Those with liver yang hyperactivity or yin vacuity patterns should consult a practitioner of Chinese medicine before using this treatment as the heat from the moxa may aggravate your condition.

For thread moxa, you will require the finest quality or grade of Japanese moxa. Pinch off a very small amount of this loose moxa and roll it lightly between your thumb and forefinger. You are aiming to make a loose, very thin thread of moxa, smaller than a grain of rice. It is important that this thread is not too large or too tightly wrapped.

Next, rub a very thin film of Tiger Balm or Temple of Heaven Balm on the point to be treated. These camphored Chinese medical salves are widely available (for suppliers, see pages 154–58). Ensure that the salve is very thinly applied. If these Chinese medicated salves are not available, then wipe the point with a tiny amount of vegetable oil or even just wet it with water. Stand the thread of moxa on end directly on the point. The oil, balm or water should provide enough stickiness to make the thread stand up. Light the thread with a thin burning incense or akabane stick. As the thread burns down towards the skin, you will feel it become warm and then hot. Remove the burning thread as soon as you feel some heat or extinguish it by pressing down on it with your finger quickly and firmly. Do not burn yourself. It is better to pull the thread off or extinguish it too soon than too late. If you do burn yourself, apply some *Ching Wan Hong* ointment. This is a Chinese burn salve, which you can buy from Chinese herbal medicine suppliers. If this is not available, try using some lavender aromatherapy oil directly on the burn this is also extremely effective.

Having extinguished the burning thread, repeat this process again. To speed up the process, you can roll a number of threads before starting the treatment. Each time the thread burns down close to the skin, extinguish it before it starts to burn you. If you do this correctly, your skin will get red and hot to the touch but you will not raise a blister. As skin texture varies from person to person, it is best to start out with three or four threads to see how you react. Increase the number of threads to between nine and 12 threads per treatment.

This treatment is especially effective for women in their late 30s and throughout their 40s whose spleen and kidney yang qi has already weakened or in older people of both sexes. It adds yang qi to the body, fortifies the spleen and invigorates the kidneys, warming yang and boosting the qi. It is best to do this treatment daily for a number of days. This can be a very beneficial home therapy for women who suffer from PMS where there are other symptoms involved such as premenstrual fatigue, loose stools, cold hands and feet, low or no libido and lower back or knee pain accompanied by frequent night-time urination that is generally copious and clear. I recommend beginning this moxibustion just before ovulation, around day 10 in the cycle. It should then be repeated every day up till the first day one of the period and then suspended. It can be done for several months in a row, but should not be done on a continual daily basis throughout the year.

There are three points which should be treated with this supplementing technique. These are: *Qi Hai* (Conception Vessel 6), *Guan Yuan* (Conception Vessel 4) and *Zu San Li* (Stomach 36).

Qi Hai is located on the midline of the body, two finger-widths below the navel. *Guan Yuan* is also located on the midline of the lower abdomen, four finger-widths below the navel.

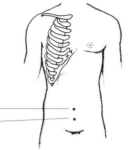

Qi Hai ————————————
Guan Yuan ——————————

Zu San Li

Zu San Li is located four finger-widths below the lower edge of the kneecap between the tibia and fibula on the outside edge of the lower leg. However, I highly recommend visiting a local professional acupuncturist so that you can be taught how to do this technique safely and effectively and shown how to locate these three points accurately.

In Chinese medicine, this technique is considered to promote longevity and good health. It is excellent for those people whose yang qi has already begun to decline due to the inevitable ageing process. It may not be beneficial for someone with ascension of hyperactive liver yang, liver fire or depressive liver heat as more heat might aggravate the situation. It is best done starting from the topmost point and moving down the body.

If there is any doubt about whether this technique is appropriate for you, please seek advice from a practitioner of Chinese medicine.

CHINESE HERBAL REMEDIES FOR HOME THERAPY

In this next section I will give you some recipes which you can make at home in the form of wines, teas and porridges. As with all Chinese herbs I strongly recommend that you seek professional guidance with regards to their usage. Should you choose to try one of these recipes and notice any unwanted side-effects, stop taking it immediately and seek professional advice.

Chinese medicinal wines

Chinese medicinal wines are part of Chinese dietary therapy. They make use of the special characteristics of alcohol as well as Chinese herbs or medicinals. Although alcohol is hot and can inflame yang heat, especially liver heat, it has the ability to move depressed qi and static blood. It can also speed up and increase the medicinal effects of herbs in the body. I recommend that you use caution should you try these recipes to improve symptoms of various patterns of headache.

For liver yang hyperactivity causing dizziness, headache, or one-sided headache, soak 200 g of Fructus Viticis *(Man Jing Zi)* in one litre of brandy or vodka for one month. Strain off the dregs and drink 1–2 tbsp of the liquid at the onset of the dizziness or headache. A slightly more elaborate formula for the same condition consists of 60 g of Fructus Viticis *(Man Jing Zi)* and 30 g each of Flos Chrysanthemi Morifolii *(Ju Hua)*, Radix Ligustici Wallichii *(Chuan Xiong)*, Radix Ledebouriellae Divaricatae *(Fang Feng)* and Herba Menthae Haplocalycis *(Bo He)*. Prepare and take this mixture in the same way as the preceding 'wine.'

For depressive liver heat or liver fire with red eyes, headache and dizziness, soak 125 g of Flos Chrysanthemi Morifolii *(Ju Hua)* in one litre of brandy or vodka for one month. Strain, discard the dregs and drink one fluid ounce of the liquid before or after dinner.

For heart blood–spleen qi vacuity, one can try either of two home-made Chinese medicinal wines. The first is made by placing 150 g of white ginseng (Radix Panacis Ginseng, *Ren Shen*) in one litre of brandy for 1–2 months. Then strain, discard the dregs, and take 1–2 fluid ounces before or after dinner. Do not use this wine if you display the signs and symptoms of depressive liver heat affecting the head and face. One can also use 150 g of Arillus Euphoriae Longanae *(Long Yan Rou)*, steeped in one litre of sake. Drink about 3 tbsp of this liquid before or after dinner each evening. Do not take this latter wine if you suffer from constipation.

For headaches due to phlegm blocking or confounding the portals of the heart, take 120 g of Rhizoma Acori Graminei *(Shi Chang Pu)* and soak this in one litre of vodka for 3–5 days. Take 10–20 ml of the resulting medicinal wine three times per day on an empty stomach.

For one-sided headache complicated by either blood vacuity or blood stasis, or as a first-aid remedy for any kind of headache, soak 90 g of Radix Ligustici Wallichii *(Chuan Xiong)* in one pint of rice wine for seven days. Drink a small cup of the liquid twice a day.

These are only a few of the Chinese medicinal wines and elixirs that can be made and used at home for the treatment of headaches. More information on Chinese medicinal wines is contained in my book *Chinese Medical Wines and Elixirs* (see page 153).

Chinese medicinal porridges

Like the Chinese medicinal wines discussed above, Chinese medicinal porridges are a specialised part of Chinese dietary therapy. Porridges are very easily digestible since they already take the form of a warm soup and so they are a particularly good way of eating nutritious grains that could otherwise be difficult to digest. Chinese medicinals cooked with grains in the form of a porridge provide a high-powered and easily assimilated nutritious 'health food' of the first order.

For wind cold headache, stir-fry till yellow 15 g of Fructus Xanthii Sibirici *(Cang Er Zi)*. Then add to 200 ml of water and boil until reduced to 100 ml of liquid. Strain, discard the dregs, add 400 ml of water and cook 50 g of rice in this herbal 'tea'. Eat the resulting porridge twice per day.

For liver fire headache, decoct 200 g of uncooked Gypsum Fibrosum *(Shi Gao)* in 300 ml of water till the liquid is reduced to 200 ml. Strain, discard the dregs and use the liquid plus another 600 ml of water to cook 100 g of rice into porridge. Eat this every day for breakfast and lunch.

For pain at the top of the head due to liver yang hyperactivity counterflowing upwards, cook 50 g of rice into porridge with water. When the porridge is half-cooked, add 3 g of powdered Fructus Evodiae Rutecarpae *(Wu Zhu Yu)* and cook until soft. Towards the end of the cooking time, add two slices of fresh ginger. Eat warm.

For headache associated with high blood pressure in turn due to liver yang hyperactivity, wash 120 g of celery and cut the stalks into pieces. Cook with 250 g of rice and water into porridge and add a little salt to taste. Eat regularly.

For headache in the elderly accompanied by dry, bound stools and constipation, mash 30 g each of Semen Pruni Persicae *(Tao Ren)* and pine nuts and 10 g of Semen Pruni (*Yu Li Ren)*. Boil this mash in water. Then add 30 g of rice and cook into porridge. Eat daily on an empty stomach.

For qi vacuity headache, cook 30 g of Radix Astragali Membranacei *(Huang Qi)* with 6 g of Pericarpium Citri Reticulatae *(Chen Pi)* in 600 ml of water for 20 minutes. Strain, discard the dregs and then use the resulting medicinal 'tea' to cook 50 g of white rice. Alternatively, take 3 g of powdered Radix Panacis Ginseng *(Ren Shen)* and cook this with 100 g of white rice in water.

Yet another option is to take 5 g of Ginseng and 20 g of powdered Sclerotium Poriae Cocos *(Fu Ling)* and cook this with 60 g of white rice in water. During the last 5–7 minutes of cooking, add two slices of fresh ginger. If you cannot find ginseng, you can use 30 g of Radix Codonopsitis Pilosulae *(Dang Shen)* cooked with 50 g of white rice in water. Remove the Codonopsis at the end and eat the resulting porridge.

For blood vacuity headache, cook 100 g of white rice with 15 g of Radix Angelicae Sinensis *(Dang Gui)* and 10 red dates (Fructus Zizyphi Jujubae, *Da Zao*). Alternatively, cook 100 g of white rice plus 10 red dates in chicken broth and eat this for dinner every evening for a number of days.

For headache due to blood and yin vacuity, use 15 g of either Semen Biota Orientalis *(Bai Zi Ren)* or Semen Ziziphi Spinosae *(Suan Zao Ren)* with 100 g of white rice and again cook with enough water to make a thin porridge or gruel.

For headache due to phlegm confounding or blocking the portals of the head, try cooking 5 g of powdered Rhizoma Acori Graminei *(Shi Chang Pu)* with 50 g of white rice in water.

See also *The Book of Jook, Chinese Medicinal Porridges: A Healthy Alternative to the Typical Western Breakfast* (see page 153).

Chinese medicinal teas

Chinese herbal teas generally consist of one or two Chinese herbal medicinals that are made into a tea and drunk throughout the day. Chinese medicinal teas are usually simpler to prepare and taste better than multi-ingredient, professionally prescribed decoctions. They can be used in addition to professionally prescribed Chinese herbs or as an adjunct to acupuncture or other Chinese therapies for headache.

For wind cold headache, take 9 g each of Folium Perillae Frutescentis *(Zi Su Ye)*, Radix Et Rhizoma Notopterygii *(Qiang Huo)* and Folium Camelliae Sinensis (*Cha Ye*) and grind into powder. Place this powder in a cup and pour in boiling water. Allow to steep for five minutes and then drink.

For wind heat headache, take 6 g each of Folium Mori Albi *(Sang Ye)*, Flos Chrysanthemi Morifolii *(Ju Hua)*, Semen Praeparatus Sojae *(Dan Dou Chi)* and pear skin. Place the herbs in a pot and cover with water. Simmer briefly, then strain and discard the dregs. Drink the brew as a tea throughout the day.

For wind damp headache, take 10 g of Herba Elsholtziae Splendentis *(Xiang Ru)* and 5 g each of Cortex Magnoliae Officinalis *(Hou Po)* and Semen Dolichoris Lablab *(Bai Bian Dou)*. Stir-fry the Dolichos until cooked and pound into pieces. Place the herbs in a vacuum flask and pour in boiling water. Seal the vacuum flask and allow to steep for one hour. Drink the resulting brew throughout the day.

For liver yang hyperactivity headache, take 10 g of Flos Chrysanthemi Morifolii *(Ju Hua)* and 15 g of Semen Cassiae Torae *(Jue Ming Zi)*. Place in a cup, pour in boiling water, and allow to steep for five minutes. Drink this freely as a tea (the above quantity will make enough for one day's supply). Another remedy is to use 10 g of Spica Prunellae Vulgaris *(Xia Ku Cao)* and 12 g of Herba Plantaginis *(Che Qian Cao)*. Place these in a cup, pour in boiling water, and allow to steep. Use this amount as one day's dose, drinking freely as a tea.

For qi vacuity headache, boil 8 g of Radix Panacis Ginseng *(Ren Shen)* for an hour or more in eight fluid ounces of water.

Drink this as a tea throughout the day. Asian speciality food stores often sell small porcelain ginseng cookers. These lidded cups may be placed in a pan of water to create a small double-cooker. The longer you cook ginseng, the more you get out of it. As a substitute for ginseng, you can use double the amount of Radix Codonopsitis Pilosulae *(Dang Shen)*. **Do not take ginseng if you suffer from hypertension or high blood pressure.**

If you suffer from blood vacuity, you can try making a tea from 5–10 pieces of Arillus Euphoriae Longanae *(Long Yan Rou)*. Place these dried fruits in a ginseng-cooker or pressure cooker and steam thoroughly. Then put them in a teacup and steep in boiling water for 10 minutes. Drink the resulting liquid as a tea. Another option is to boil 10 pieces of Fructus Zizyphi Jujubae *(Da Zao)* in water until the fruit are thoroughly cooked and completely soft. Then use the resulting liquid to steep 5 g of green tea. Drink this as a tea any time throughout the day.

For yin and blood vacuity headache, boil 15 g of Fructus Mori Albi *(Sang Zhen)* in water. Strain, discard the dregs and drink the liquid as a daily dose. Another option is to grind into powder equal amounts of Fructus Schisandrae Chinensis *(Wu Wei Zi)* and Fructus Lycii Chinensis *(Gou Qi Zi)*. Then steep 5 g of this powder in boiling water for 10 minutes and drink as a tea throughout the day. Alternatively, use 9 g of Semen Zizyphi Spinosae *(Suan Zao Ren)*. Pound into pieces, steep in boiling water for 10 minutes, and drink throughout the day.

For phlegm obstruction, grind 6 g of Rhizoma Acori Graminei *(Shi Chang Pu)*, 6 g of Flos Jasmini *(Mo Li Hua)* and 10 g of green tea into coarse powder. Soak some of this powder in boiling water and drink as a tea any time throughout the day. (You can also use jasmine tea bought at an Asian speciality food shop.) The quantities given are for a one day's supply. Another formula for phlegm obstruction consists of

10 g of Dens Draconis *(Long Chi)* and 3 g of Rhizoma Acori Graminei *(Shi Chang Pu).* First boil the Dens Draconis in water for 10 minutes. Then add the Rhizoma Acori Graminei and continue boiling for another 10–15 minutes. Remove the dregs and drink throughout the day. You may drink up to twice the quantity prescribed per day.

For blood stasis headache or the first-aid treatment of any kind of headache, boil 3 g of Radix Ligustici Wallichii *(Chuan Xiong)* and 6 g of green tea in 300 ml of water until reduced to 150 ml of liquid. Drink this warm when there is pain or before meals, up to twice the given quantity per day.

More information on Chinese medicinal teas is given in Zong Xiao-fan and Gary Liscum's *Chinese Medicinal Teas: Simple, Proven, Folk Formulas for Common Diseases and Promoting Health* (see page 153).

HYDROTHERAPY

Hydrotherapy means water therapy and is also a part of traditional Chinese medicine. There are numerous different water treatments for helping relieve either stress in general or headaches in particular. First, begin with a warm bath. Soaking in a warm bath just slightly higher than body temperature for 15–20 minutes can free and smooth the flow of qi and blood and relieve premenstrual tension and irritability. It can also calm the spirit and hasten sleep. Taking a warm bath a half hour before going to bed can help insomnia.

However, when using a warm bath, do be careful not to use water so hot or to stay in the bath so long that sweat breaks out on your forehead. We lose yang qi as well as body fluids when we sweat. Because fluids and blood share a common source, excessive sweating can cause problems for women with blood and yin vacuities. Sweating can also worsen yang qi vacuities in people whose spleen and kidneys are weak. So, unless given a specific hot bath prescription from your Chinese medical practitioner, I recommend you do not stay in warm baths until you sweat. Although you may feel pleasantly relaxed at first, you may later feel excessively fatigued or hot and thirsty. In menopausal women, hot baths may increase hot flushes and night sweats.

If, due to depression transforming heat, yang qi is exuberant and counterflowing upwards, it may cause migraines and tension headaches, hot flushes, night sweats, painful, red eyes and even nosebleeds. To relieve these symptoms, place your feet in cold water up to your ankles for 15–20 minutes at a time. You may also soak your hands in cold water or put cold, wet compresses on the back of your neck. The first two treatments seek to draw yang qi away from the head either to the lower part of the body or out to the extremities. The third treatment seeks to block and stop yang qi from counterflowing upwards, causing congestion and damaging the blood vessels in the head.

People who catch cold easily or who are struggling with obesity can use cool baths, slightly lower than body temperature, for 10 minutes per day. Although this may seem contradictory, since cold is yin and these patients already suffer from a yang insufficiency, this brief and not too extreme exposure to cool water stimulates the body to produce more yang qi. In Chinese medicine, it is not advisable to take cold baths during menstruation as this may retard the free flow of qi and blood and lead to dysmenorrhoea (painful menstruation).

CREATING A PERSONALISED REGIME

You do not need to do each and every one of these home treatments for every case of headache. Choose several of them that appeal to you and are manageable. The more severe your headache symptoms the more support you are likely to need. It is best to make sure you are using the three free therapies and then add these home remedies whichever you can best manage. Chinese self-massage and seven star hammering are rather time-consuming, but they are very effective therapies.

Given the wide choice of Chinese self-therapies in this chapter, it should be possible for you to find the materials or the time to put at least one of these into practice. In less severe cases of infrequent headaches, that may be all that is required, but in more difficult, stubborn cases, you may have to use two or three of the therapies to ensure lasting relief from head and face pain.

CHINESE MEDICAL RESEARCH ON HEADACHES

his chapter contains some recently published reports on research done in the People's Republic of China on the Chinese medical treatment of headaches. The first five deal with Chinese herbal medicine and the sixth deals with acupuncture. The last one discusses the combined treatment of neurovascular diseases with both acupuncture and Chinese herbs. There are approximately 20 provinces in the People's Republic of China and each province publishes a monthly provincial Chinese medical journal. In addition, each province has a provincial Chinese medical college. Many of these colleges also publish a monthly Chinese medical journal. This means that there are 30 or more Chinese medical journals published each month in China with 40–60 articles per issue of each journal. There are thousands of research reports on the efficacy of Chinese medicine published each year.

As the reader will see, the reports here describe what is called a clinical audit. A number of patients were given a certain treatment; they were then followed up to see how the treatment worked in terms of their major complaint. The patients in this study had chosen to be treated with Chinese medicine and both they and the doctors in this study were fully cognisant of what they were doing. This means that this study was not either single-blind or double-blind. Patient's responses were not compared to either a placebo or other comparison treatment. The sole interest in this research was to monitor a self-selected group of headache sufferers when treated with a particular Chinese medicine protocol which they knew they were taking and chose to receive.

This is called outcome-based research and it mirrors real-life practice. It is not an artificial construct seeking to rule out all possible co-factors, such as practitioner and/or patient belief. This type of research is becoming more and more accepted in the Western scientific community as Western researchers are beginning to understand the limitations and fallacies, not to mention the cost, of prospective, double-blind, placebo-controlled research. Double-blind, placebo-controlled research was instituted in the 1960s after the thalidomide disaster and quickly became the gold standard of medical research. However, such research does not mimic real-life clinical practice where patients knowingly select their care providers and knowingly select the type of treatment they want, such as standard Western drug therapy, nutritional therapy, acupuncture, or herbal medicine.

As Western researchers move more and more towards outcome-based research and away from the cost and artificiality of the double-blind, placebo-controlled, prospective study, they will also come to realise that there is a veritable mountain of such outcome-based research on the safety and efficacy of Chinese medicine in the Chinese medical journals published over the last 40 years in the People's Republic of China.

'A Report on the Treatment of 86 Cases of Recalcitrant Headache with *Dang Gui Si Ni Tang Jia Jian*' by Jin Shao-xian and Zong Hui-min, appearing in *Tian Jin Zhong Yi* (Tianjin Chinese Medicine), No. 6, 1993
This clinical audit discusses the treatment of 86 cases of recalcitrant headache with *Dang Gui Si Ni Tang Jia Jian* (Dang Gui Four Counterflows Decoction with Additions and Subtractions). Of the 86 cases, 74 were outpatients and 12 were hospitalised with 27 (34 per cent) being men and 59 (66 per cent) women. Their ages ranged from 12 to 74 years of age. Nine cases were aged between 12 and 20, 26 between 20 and

30, 18 between 31 and 40, 21 between 41 and 50, 7 between 50 and 60, four between 61 and 70, and one case was 74 years old. The course of suffering had lasted from a few days to several months in 28 cases, 1–5 years in 32 cases, 5–10 years in 21 cases, 10–20 years in 11 cases, and over 20 years in four cases. Western medical diagnosis ruled out that these patients' headaches were due to cervical vertebrae disease, brain tumours, brain abscess, nose or throat cancer, swelling of the eye socket or retention of inner ear fluid.

Based on Chinese medical pattern discrimination, these patients' headaches were categorised as external invasion and internal injury. Their symptoms included hands and feet that were chilly, an ashen complexion, cold sweating, hiccups, vomiting of foamy saliva, and a fine, weak pulse or fine pulse on the verge of stopping. According to Chinese medical pattern discrimination, these signs and symptoms are categorised as blood vacuity cold pattern, with static blood obstructing and checking the channels and vessels. According to the author this type of recalcitrant headache is due to wind cold evils entering the channels and vessels where they obstruct the clear yang qi. The qi and blood become static and stagnant and this obstructs and checks the vessels and pathways. Thus the qi and blood of the clear portals counterflow chaotically and this produces headaches. If evil qi is retained, it may hide for a long time and not be removed. This results in a long period of suffering and difficulty curing this condition. The fact that the hands and feet suffer inversion chill and the pulse is fine and on the verge of ceasing clarifies that this disease should mostly be categorised as blood vacuity, cold stasis.

Dang Gui Si Ni Tang Jia Jian was administered, consisting of:

15 g Radix Angelicae Sinensis *(Dang Gui)*
 3 g Herba Asari Cum Radice *(Xi Xin)*

6 g   Medulla Tetrapanacis Papyriferi *(Tong Cao)*
5 g   Fructus Evodiae Rutecarpae *(Wu Zhu Yu)*
10 g Ramulus Cinnamomi Cassiae *(Gui Zhi)*
12 g Radix Albus Paeoniae Lactiflorae *(Bai Shao)*
12 g Mix-fried Radix Glycyrrhizae *(Gan Cao)*
10 g Fructus Zizyphi Jujubae *(Da Zao)*
12 g Uncooked Rhizoma Zingiberis *(Sheng Jiang)*

This quantity was given per day during headache attacks. Once the headache was relaxed and resolved, administration was stopped. In between episodes, it is also acceptable to use double the amount of the above formula made into honey pills. In this case, one can take 10 g of such pills 2–3 times per day. If there is repeated occurrence of headache, one can then take this formula as a decoction.

If wind cold was more in evidence, then Radix Et Rhizoma Notopterygii *(Qiang Huo)* and Radix Ligustici Wallichii *(Chuan Xiong)* were added. If wind heat was more apparent, Herba Menthae Haplocalycis *(Bo He)*, Flos Chrysanthemi Morifolii *(Ju Hua)*, and uncooked Gypsum Fibrosum *(Shi Gao)* were added. For wind dampness, Rhizoma Atractylodis *(Cang Zhu)* and Radix Angelicae Dahuricae *(Bai Zhi)* were added. If there was more qi vacuity, Radix Panacis Ginseng *(Ren Shen)* and Radix Astragali Membranacei *(Huang Qi)* were added. For blood vacuity, Radix Polygoni Multiflori *(Shou Wu)* was added and Radix Angelicae Sinensis *(Dang Gui)* and Radix Albus Paeoniae Lactiflorae *(Bai Shao)* were doubled. If kidney vacuity was apparent, Fructus Corni Officinalis *(Shan Zhu)*, Fructus Lycii Chinensis *(Gou Qi)* and Plastrum Testudinis *(Gui Ban)* were added. For phlegm dampness, *Er Chen Tang* (Two Aged Ingredients Decoction) was added. If there was liver yang hyperactivity, Cinnamomum and Evodia were subtracted and Fructus Gardeniae Jasminoidis *(Zhi Zi)*, Radix Gentianae Scabrae *(Long Dan Cao)*, Ramulus Uncariae Cum

Uncis *(Gou Teng)* and Bombyx Batryticatus *(Tian Chong)* were added.

Of the 86 patients treated with this protocol, 31 (36.1 per cent) were cured, 29 (33.7 per cent) obviously improved, 21 (24.5 per cent) experienced some improvement, and five (5.7 per cent) experienced no improvement. Thus the overall effectiveness rate was 94.3 per cent.

Case history

The patient was a 28-year-old, unmarried servicewoman who typically had irregular and painful periods. Because of work-related problems, she became excessively exhausted. She developed depression and became unable to relax, which led to her not being able to fall asleep at night. One week after her period, she experienced dizziness and blurred vision accompanied by almost unbearable piercing pain at the crown of her head. She also vomited clear fluid. After she had taken some pain-relievers and muscle-relaxants, her pain stopped. One month later, during her period, she got the same headache as before. After this, every month during her period she would get the same headache. Her pulse was fine, weak and forceless. Her tongue was pale with a thin, white, moist coating. She was given *Dang Gui Si Ni Jia Wu Zhu Yu Sheng Jiang Tang* (Dang Gui Four Counterflows plus Evodia and Uncooked Ginger Decoction):

10 g   Fructus Evodiae Rutecarpae *(Wu Zhu)*
 5 g   Uncooked Rhizoma Zingiberis *(Sheng Jiang)*
 5 g   Fructus Zizyphi Jujubae *(Da Zao)*
10 g   Ramulus Cinnamomi Cassiae *(Gui Zhi)*
12 g   Radix Albus Paeoniae Lactiflorae *(Bai Shao)*
10 g   Mix-fried Radix Glycyrrhizae *(Gan Cao)*
 5 g   Herba Asari Cum Radice *(Xi Xin)*
15 g   Radix Angelicae Sinensis *(Dang Gui)*
 6 g   Medullae Tetrapanacis Papyriferi *(Tong Cao)*

After 30 doses of this formula, there was no further recurrence of the headache and, on follow-up six months later, the headache had been completely cured.

'The Treatment of 52 Cases of Recalcitrant Migraines with *Huo Xue Hua Yu Xiao Tong Tang*' by Wang Xian-qi and Sun Qing, *Xin Zhong Yi* (New Chinese Medicine), No. 7, 1996
This article reports on the treatment of 52 cases of recalcitrant migraine headache with the self-composed formula, *Huo Xue Hua Yu Xiao Tong Tang* (Quicken the Blood, Transform Stasis and Disperse Pain Decoction). All 52 of these patients had previously taken Western medicine for a long time without being cured. Among them, there were 20 men and 32 women. Their ages ranged from 15 to 55 years old. Five cases were 20 years of age or less, 22 were 21–30, 14 cases were 31–40, seven cases were 41–50, and four cases were over 50 years of age. The shortest course of suffering was one year and the longest was 23 years.

Treatment consisted of the following formula:

15 g   Radix Angelicae Sinensis *(Dang Gui)*
15 g   Radix Bupleuri *(Chai Hu)*
15 g   Radix Angelicae Dahuricae *(Bai Zhi)*
15 g   Radix Et Rhizoma Notopterygii *(Qiang Huo)*
15 g   Radix Ledebouriellae Divaricatae *(Fang Feng)*
15 g   Radix Ligustici Wallichii *(Chuan Xiong)*
10 g   Semen Pruni Persicae *(Tao Ren)*
10 g   Flos Carthami Tinctorii *(Hong Hua)*
10 g   Radix Scutellariae Baicalensis *(Huang Qin)*
10 g   Rhizoma Coptidis Chinensis *(Huang Lian)*
10 g   Mix-fried Radix Glycyrrhizae *(Gan Cao)*

If there was accompanying insomnia, 10 g of Semen Zizyphi Spinosae *(Suan Zao Ren)* and 15 g of Rhizoma Acori Graminei *(Shi Chang Pu)* were added. The above medicinals were decocted in water twice. Then 500 ml of the resulting liquid was drunk warm every morning and evening. Six days equalled one course of therapy. Between each course, there were two days of rest when the herbs were not taken. The shortest course of treatment was one course of therapy, while the longest was five courses.

Cure was defined as complete disappearance of all the symptoms with no recurrence on follow-up after six months. Based on this definition, 36 cases were judged cured and 13 cases improved, meaning that their headaches had for the most part disappeared. However, if they became emotionally upset or overworked and fatigued, they did have recurrences. Happily, these recurrences were very slight. Three cases had no relief by using the above protocol. This meant that there was no change for the better in their symptoms from before to after treatment with this formula. Therefore, the overall effectiveness rate of this protocol was 94.2 per cent.

'Experiences in the Treatment of 36 Cases of Migraines with *Xiong Qi Shao Zhi Tang'* by Huang Cheng-yun, appearing in *Hei Long Jiang Zhong Yi Yao (Heilongjiang Chinese Medicine and Medicinals)*, No. 5, 1996

In this study of 36 cases of migraine headache, ten patients were men and 26 patients were women. The youngest was 16 and the oldest was 71 years old. Four cases were aged 16–20, 16 were 21–30, nine were 31–40, five were 41–50, and 12 cases were over 50 years of age. Twelve cases had been sick for one year or less, 14 cases for 1–2 years, six cases for 3–5 years, and four cases for more than five years. In terms of frequency of attacks, 15 cases had at least one attack per month, while 21 cases had one or two migraines each year.

One-sided headaches occurred in 16 cases, while 12 cases had bilateral head pain. Another eight cases had one-sided and crown-of-the-head pain. Throbbing pain affected 30 cases, five had visual disturbances, 32 had prodromal auras that appeared as a warning before the other symptoms, and 22 had family histories of migraines. Most of the women reported that their headaches had started around puberty.

The treatment consisted of self-composed *Xiong Qi Shao Zhi Tang* (Ligusticum, Pseudoginseng, Peony and Angelica Decoction). This consisted of:

15 g   Radix Ligustici Wallichii *(Chuan Xiong)*
30 g   Radix Albus Paeoniae Lactiflorae *(Bai Shao)*
12 g   Radix Angelicae Dahuricae *(Bai Zhi)*
 6 g   Radix Pseudoginseng *(San Qi)*
10 g   Flos Chrysanthemi Morifolii *(Ju Hua)*
10 g   Fructus Viticis *(Man Jing Zi)*
20 g   Uncooked Radix Rehmanniae *(Sheng Di)*
 6 g   Bombyx Batryticatus *(Jiang Can)*
10 g   Lumbricus *(Di Long)*
 6 g   Radix Glycyrrhizae *(Gan Cao)*

One quantity of these medicinals was decocted in water per day and administered warm in divided doses.

This formula was modified for individual differences. If there was a wind heat pattern, 30 g of uncooked Gypsum Fibrosum *(Shi Gao)* and 6 g of Folium Bambusae *(Zhu Ye)* were added. If there was a wind cold pattern, 10 g of Herba Seu Flos Schizonepetae Tenuifoliae *(Jing Jie Sui)* and 5 g of Herba Asari Cum Radice *(Xi Xin)* were added. If there was insomnia, 30 g each of uncooked Concha Ostreae *(Mu Li)* and Os Draconis *(Long Gu)* were added as well as 20 g of Caulis Polygoni Multiflori *(Ye Jiao Teng)*.[3] If there was constipation, then 6–10 g of Radix Et Rhizoma Rhei *(Da Huang)* were added. If

---

[3] It is interesting to note that Western researchers are now beginning to understand that curing sleep disorders can have a therapeutic effect on chronic headaches. Chinese medicine treats insomnia quite well without the use of sedatives which cause grogginess the next day.

there was heart vexation and easy anger, 10 g each of Radix Bupleuri *(Chai Hu)* and Radix Scutellariae Baicalensis *(Huang Qin)* were added. If there was nausea and vomiting, 10 g of Rhizoma Pinelliae Ternatae *(Ban Xia)* and 12 g of Caulis Bambusae In Taeniis *(Zhu Ru)* were added. If there was pain at the crown of the head, 15 g of Radix Et Rhizoma Ligustici Sinensis *(Gao Ben)* were added. If there were visual disturbances, 15 g of Fructus Lycii Chinensis *(Gou Qi Zi)* were added. And if there was high blood pressure, 12 g of Spica Prunellae Vulgaris *(Xia Ku Cao)* and 15 g of Radix Achyranthis Bidentatae *(Huai Niu Xi)* were added.

Complete cure was defined as cessation of headache attacks with no recurrence on follow-up after two years. Improvement meant that the number of attacks was markedly decreased and the symptoms were markedly diminished. No cure meant that there was no change in the headaches or that they got worse. Based on these criteria, 24 cases were cured and 12 cases were improved. Ten cases took a turn for the better within three days, 16 improved within seven, and ten cases improved within 20 days.

The author of this protocol based the composition of the formula on Ye Tian-shi's statements: 'Initially diseases are in the channels, while enduring disease enters the network vessels since the channels govern the qi and the network vessels govern the blood. Thus one can know when one must treat the qi and when one must treat the blood.' Because migraines tend to be an enduring, long-lasting condition, Dr Huang feels that the emphasis in their treatment should be on quickening the blood and transforming stasis. However, this formula does also dispel wind, nourish yin and clear heat. In addition, it includes several medicinals that are known to be antispasmodic, thus relieving the constriction of the blood vessels that is associated with migraines.

'An Analysis of the Treatment Efficacy of *Qing Shang Quan Tong Tang* **on Vascular Headaches' by Zhang Yue-mei and Fang Dong,** *Hei Long Jiang Zhong Yi Yao (Heilongjiang Chinese Medicine and Medicinals)***, No. 2, 1995**

Between January 1992 and April 1994, the author of this study treated 34 patients with vascular headaches with *Qing Shang Quan Tong Tang* (Clear the Upper and Purify Pain Decoction). Eight of the patients in this study were men and 26 were women. The youngest was 17 and the oldest was 61. Six were aged 17–25, 11 were 26–35, nine were 36–45, six were 46–55, and two were over 55 years of age. The shortest course of suffering was seven months and the longest was nine years. Eight cases had been ill for one year or less, 16 had been suffering from headaches for 1–5 years, and ten cases had been suffering for 6–9 years.

Four cases had pain mainly on the left side of the forehead. Six cases had pain mainly on the right side of the forehead. Left-sided temporal pain affected 11 cases and nine cases had right-sided temporal pain. Four cases had bilateral forehead pain. In 25 cases, the pain was throbbing, while in nine cases it was distended pain. Nine cases also had dizziness and vertigo at the time of occurrence, while 17 had nausea and vomiting.

Qing Shang Quan Tong Tang consisted of:

12–15 g	Radix Angelicae Sinensis *(Dang Gui)*
12–15 g	Radix Ligustici Wallichii *(Chuan Xiong)*
9–12 g	Radix Angelicae Dahuricae *(Bai Zhi)*
2–3 g	Herba Asari Cum Radice *(Xi Xin)*
9–12 g	Radix Et Rhizoma Notopterygii *(Qiang Huo)*
9–12 g	Radix Angelicae Pubescentis *(Du Huo)*
6–10 g	Fructus Viticis *(Man Jing Zi)*
9–12 g	Rhizoma Atractylodis *(Cang Zhu)*
10–12 g	Tuber Ophiopogonis Japonici *(Mai Dong)*
12–15 g	Radix Scutellariae Baicalensis *(Huang Qin)*

12–15 g	Flos Chrysanthemi Morifolii (Ju Hua)
9–12 g	Radix Ledebouriellae Divaricatae (Fang Feng)
6–9 g	Radix Glycyrrhizae (Gan Cao)
3 slices	Uncooked Rhizoma Zingiberis (Sheng Jiang)

Individualised modifications were added as follows: if there was accompanying dizziness and vertigo, 15–24 g of Rhizoma Alismatis (Ze Xie) and 15–24 g of Rhizoma Atractylodis Macrocephalae (Bai Zhu) were added. If there was nausea and vomiting, 9–15 g of ginger-processed Caulis Bambusae In Taeniis (Zhu Ru) and 9–12 g of Rhizoma Pinelliae Ternatae (Ban Xia) were added. If there was a bitter taste in the mouth, red eyes and constipation with yellow tongue fur, 9–12 g of Radix Et Rhizoma Rhei (Da Huang) and 9–12 g of Fructus Immaturus Citri Aurantii (Zhi Shi) were added. One quantity of the above formula was decocted in water and administered each day, with ten days equalling one course of therapy.

Cure meant that the headaches disappeared and there was no recurrence on follow-up after one year. Marked effect was defined as the disappearance of the headaches after treatment, some recurrence on follow-up, but markedly decreased pain and fewer attacks; when these medicinals were given again, they were able to eliminate the headaches. Some effect meant that the aching and pain reduced but were not completely eliminated. No effect meant that there was no change for the better after two courses of therapy. Based on these criteria, 23 cases were cured, seven cases had a marked effect, three cases received some effect, and two cases had no effect. Therefore, the overall effectiveness rate was 94.2 per cent.

Case history

The patient was a 38-year-old female who came for her first examination on February 21 1992. She had had migraine headaches for seven years. She had had several EEGS which were all normal. Hospital doctors had diagnosed her as suffering from vascular headaches. She had taken several types of Western medicine but with only very little effect. For the last ten days, due to work stress, she had been having throbbing, left-sided forehead pain. She complained of photophobia (aversion to light) and she was afraid to move. The pain was almost unbearable at times, and she could not go to sleep at night. The attacks were accompanied by nausea and vomiting. Her tongue was dark with thin, white fur, while her pulse was bowstring and tight.

Based on the above signs and symptoms, her Chinese medical pattern discrimination was categorised as external wind internally invading. The channel qi, therefore, was inhibited and the network vessels were not freely flowing. The qi and blood was static and stagnant. She was prescribed *Qing Shang Quan Tong Tang* with added ingredients. The prescription read:

12 g	Radix Angelicae Sinensis *(Dang Gui)*
15 g	Radix Ligustici Wallichii *(Chuan Xiong)*
10 g	Radix Et Rhizoma Notopterygii *(Qiang Huo)*
9 g	Radix Angelicae Pubescentis *(Du Huo)*
9 g	Rhizoma Atractylodis *(Cang Zhu)*
12 g	Radix Ledebouriellae Divaricatae *(Fang Feng)*
3 g	Herba Asari Cum Radice *(Xi Xin)*
3 g	Fructus Viticis *(Man Jing Zi)*
12 g	Flos Chrysanthemi Morifolii *(Ju Hua)*
12 g	Tuber Ophiopogonis Japonici *(Mai Dong)*
10 g	Radix Angelicae Dahuricae *(Bai Zhi)*
10 g	Radix Scutellariae Baicalensis *(Huang Qin)*
9 g	Radix Glycyrrhizae *(Gan Cao)*
10 g	Ginger-processed Caulis Bambusae In Taeniis *(Zhu Ru)*
10 g	Rhizoma Pinelliae Ternatae *(Ban Xia)*
3 slices	Uncooked Rhizoma Zingiberis *(Sheng Jiang)*

After she had taken three quantities of this formula, the aching and pain had obviously diminished. Then another three quantities of the same formula were given. At the end of that time, all her symptoms had completely disappeared. In order to consolidate the therapeutic effect, another three quantities of the same herbs were given. After taking these, she then stopped taking any Chinese medicinals. On follow-up after two years, there had been no recurrence.

'The Treatment of 64 Cases of Static Blood Headache with Self-composed *Zhu Yu Zhi Tong Tang*' by Sun Hai-long *et al.*, appearing in *Hei Long Jiang Zhong Yi Yao (Heilongjiang Chinese Medicine and Medicinals)*, No. 4, 1995
The 64 patients described in this study were seen between 1985 and 1993. All suffered from chronic headaches which felt piercing or stabbing. Their tongues were purple and dark and their pulses were bowstring or fine and choppy. Therefore, all were categorised as suffering from blood stasis pattern headaches. Amongst this group, there were 38 men and 26 women. The oldest was 52 and the youngest was 15 years old. Most of the patients were between 40 and 50 years of age.

Self-composed *Zhu Yu Zhi Tong Tang* (Dispel Stasis and Stop Pain Decoction) was composed of:

30 g   Radix Ligustici Wallichii *(Chuan Xiong)*
15 g   Radix Salviae Miltiorrhizae *(Dan Shen)*
10 g   Semen Pruni Persicae *(Tao Ren)*
10 g   Flos Carthami Tinctorii *(Hong Hua)*
10 g   Radix Rubrus Paeoniae Lactiflorae *(Chi Shao)*
 5 g   Radix Pseudoginseng *(San Qi)*
2 strips Scolopendra Subspinipes *(Wu Gong)*
10 g   Rhizoma Acori Graminei *(Shi Chang Pu)*

These were decocted in water and administered, one quantity per day, taken warm, morning and night.

Complete cure meant that the headaches disappeared. Improvement meant that the head pain diminished, their duration was shorter, and the time between episodes was longer. No effect meant that there was no change in the symptoms of headache. Based on these definitions, 40 cases were judged cured, 22 improved, and only two cases felt no effect. Therefore, the overall effectiveness rate for this protocol was 96 per cent.

'The Acupuncture Treatment of 65 Cases of Migraines' by Bai Hui-min, appearing in *Tian Jin Zhong Yi Xue Yuan Xue Bao (The Journal of the Tian Jin College of Chinese Medicine)*, No. 2, 1996
The author begins by stating that one-sided headache (the term most commonly used for migraines in Chinese medicine) is a type of recurrent vascular headache. It is commonly accompanied by nausea and vomiting. The author of this study has been treating this kind of headache for many years with two acupuncture points.

Of the 65 cases 22 (33.8 per cent) were men, while 43 (66.2 per cent) were women. The oldest patient was 57 and the youngest was 15. The longest course of suffering was 30 years and the shortest was three months. In 28 cases, the aching and pain occurred on the left side. In 30 cases, it occurred on the right side and in another seven cases, it was bilateral. CT scan and other modern Western diagnostic methods were used to rule out other diagnoses. During this study, previously used Chinese and Western medications were stopped.

The treatment method consisted of two points: *Feng Chi* (Gall Bladder 20) and *Qiu Xu* (Gall Bladder 40). After disinfecting the areas to be stimulated, the needles were inserted at these two points and then manipulated with draining technique. (This is the technique for draining off replete evils.) The needles were then retained for 20 minutes.

During this time, they were manipulated twice. One treatment was given every other day, and ten treatments constituted one course of therapy.

Cure was defined as complete disappearance of all symptoms with no recurrence within one year. Marked effect was defined as a marked improvement in the symptoms, still with slight headaches. Some effect meant that the area affected by the pain was smaller and that the degree of pain was less. No effect meant that there was no improvement after the treatment.

Based on these criteria, 22 cases (33.9 per cent) were cured, 29 cases (44.6 per cent) registered marked effect, 11 cases (16.9 per cent) got some effect, and three cases (4.6 per cent) felt no effect. Thus the overall effectiveness rate was 95.3 per cent.

Case history

The patient was a 41-year-old woman who worked as an engineering teacher. She was first seen on September 12 1992. She had had recurrent right-sided headaches for eight years. Often, the attacks occurred when she was overworked or when she was emotionally stressed. When the pain was severe, it was accompanied by ringing in the ears, blurred vision, nausea and a desire to vomit. She had already tried Western medicine without effect. Neurological examination was negative. X-rays of the vertebrae in her neck and a CT scan of her brain showed no abnormalities. She was, therefore, diagnosed as suffering from migraine headaches.

Treatment consisted of manipulating needles at the two points of *Feng Chi* and *Qiu Xu*. After the first treatment, the head pain had markedly decreased. At night, she no longer had to take sedatives and analgesics in order to go to sleep. After the third treatment, the headache was greatly diminished and extra fatigue from work did not aggravate it.

After ten treatments, the symptoms had all disappeared and she was judged cured. On follow-up after one year, her headaches had not returned.

In the author's discussion of this study, one-sided pain is categorised in Chinese medicine as *shao yang* channel head pain. *Feng Chi* and *Qiu Xu* are both points on the foot *shao yang* gall bladder channel. *Feng Chi* is located on the head. It is able to course and free the flow of the channels and network vessels. Further, it dispels wind and stops pain. It is an essential point in the treatment of headache. It is mentioned as a remedy for headache in such early Chinese acupuncture classics as *Zhen Jiu Jia Yi Jing (The Systematic Classic of Acupuncture and Moxibustion)* and *Zhen Jiu Da Cheng (The Great Compendium of Acupuncture and Moxibustion)*. *Qiu Xu* is the so-called source point on the gall bladder channel. That means it treats diseases of both the viscera (i.e. liver) and the bowels (i.e. gall bladder). Although it is located on the foot, it is recorded in the *Ling Shu (Spiritual Pivot)* that: 'For diseases of the head, choose the foot.' This has since become known as the acupuncture principle of treating points below for diseases above and vice versa. These two points are combined together based on the principle of choosing points above and below on the affected channel.

'The Treatment of 30 Cases of Neurovascular Headache with Acupuncture and Chinese Herbs' by Li Che-cheng and Xu Hui-min, appearing in *Hei Long Jiang Zhong Yi Yao (Heilongjiang Chinese Medicine and Medicinals)*, No. 1, 1996
Beginning in 1990, the author of this article treated 30 cases of neurovascular headache with a combination of acupuncture and Chinese herbal medicine. Of these patients, 12 were men and 18 were women. They ranged in age from 12 to 61 years old, while their condition had lasted from two weeks to 18 years. In 18 cases, headaches had been occurring for more

than one year. In most cases, the number of attacks were numerous and frequent. In two cases, attacks occurred three times or more each day. In 18 cases, they occurred once or twice each day. Another eight cases had headaches once between one and three times per week, while another two cases had headaches once every 1–2 weeks. In 21 cases, the pain was one-sided, and in nine cases it was bilateral. All the patients were diagnosed by Western medical means as suffering from neurovascular headaches. There was a connection between the occurrence of these headaches and changes in emotions and/or sleep patterns. The pain was mostly very severe and lasted from several minutes to several hours. If the headache was severe, it was typically accompanied by sweating, heart palpitations, nausea and vomiting.

The Chinese herbal formula consisted of:

60 g   Radix Angelicae Dahuricae *(Bai Zhi)*
30 g   Radix Ligustici Wallichii *(Chuan Xiong)*
30 g   Cortex Albizziae Julibrissin *(He Huan Pi)*
30 g   Radix Glycyrrhizae *(Gan Cao)*

These quantities were ground into fine powder and divided into 20 doses. Each morning and evening, the patients in this study took one dose mixed in water.

The acupuncture consisted of manipulating needles at *Tai Yang* (extra channel), *Shuai Gu* (Gall Bladder 8), and *Bai Hui* (Governing Vessel 20). Each of these points was stimulated with even draining/even supplementing hand technique and the needles were retained for 30 minutes. This was done once each day.

Every person in this study registered a marked effect. After continuous treatment for 3–6 days, the headaches had either disappeared or decreased in frequency or duration. In all, 19 patients (63.3 per cent) were completely cured. This meant that their symptoms disappeared, their EEG was normal, and that neurological tests were negative. The other 11 cases (36.7 per cent) all improved. Their headaches disappeared. However, if they overworked or experienced emotional tension, they did feel a very slight degree of aching and pain. The authors of this study say that, in their experience, most neurovascular headaches have to do with a combination of wind and blood stasis. Therefore, this treatment aims to dispel wind and stop pain, quicken the blood and move stasis.

As stated earlier, I have abstracted these clinical audits on the effectiveness of Chinese medicine and acupuncture from various Chinese medical journals at random – I went to my bookshelf and pulled down a handful of issues of a couple of different journals and this is what I found. It is only a small fraction of the Chinese research on all types of headaches published in such Chinese journals in the last 40 years.

Personally, when I read these reports, as a clinician, I think they look quite convincing. The protocols described did not necessarily cure every single patient, but typically 90 per cent or more got some benefit. Those are pretty good odds. If you agree with me, then you might consider trying Chinese medicine and/or acupuncture for your headaches, be they migraine, tension, cluster or sinus headaches.

FINDING A PRACTITIONER OF CHINESE MEDICINE

Chinese medicine is one of the fastest growing holistic health care systems in the West today. In the UK there are at least ten colleges offering professional training courses in acupuncture, moxibustion, Chinese herbal medicine and Chinese medical massage; some offer a university degree. In addition, many of the graduates of these courses have done postgraduate studies at colleges and hospitals in China, Taiwan, Hong Kong and Japan. A growing number of trained Oriental medical practitioners have emigrated from China, Japan and Korea to practise acupuncture and Chinese herbal medicine in the West.

Chinese medicine, including acupuncture, is a discrete and independent health care profession. It is not simply a technique that can easily be added to the array of techniques of some other health care profession. The study of Chinese medicine, acupuncture and Chinese herbs is as rigorous as is the study of allopathic, chiropractic, naturopathic or homoeopathic medicine. Previous training in any one of these other systems does not automatically confer competence or knowledge in Chinese medicine. In order to get the full benefits and ensure the safety of Chinese medicine, it is best to seek out professionally trained and qualified practitioners.

When seeking a qualified and knowledgeable practitioner, personal recommendations are often the best method. It is essential to work with a practitioner who communicates effectively enough for the patient to feel understood. Here are some questions you might ask when selecting a practitioner:
- Where did you qualify and are you a member of the appropriate professional body ?
- What is your experience in treating my condition?

- Do you use disposable needles?
- How often will I need to see you and for how many visits?
- How much do you charge?

Many practitioners will be happy to talk on the phone or offer a short introductory consultation so that you can assess whether you will feel comfortable working with them.

Below is a list of professional bodies for Chinese medicine in the UK. I have included information on shiatsu practitioners as it can be a very effective therapy to treat headaches.

Acupuncture
The British Acupuncture Council
63 Jeddo Road
London
W12 9HQ
Tel: 020 8735 0400
Fax: 020 8735 0404
E-mail: infor@acupuncture.org.uk
Website: www.acupuncture.org.uk

Members have the initials: MBAcC.

Chinese herbal medicine
The Register of Chinese Herbal Medicine
PO Box 400
Wembley
Middlesex
HA9 9NZ
Tel/fax: 07000 790332
Website: www.rchm.co.uk

Members have the initials: MRCHM.

Japanese herbal medicine
The Kanpo Association
9a Ingatestone Road
Brentwood
Essex
CM15 8AP
Tel: 01277 260080

Members have the initials: KANPO.
Members of the Kanpo Association are not bound by a code of ethics and practice or covered by insurance unless they also belong to another professional body. Most practitioners of kanpo belong to one of the three other professional bodies.

Shiatsu
The Shiatsu Society UK
Barber House
Storeys Bar Road
Fengate
Peterborough
PE1 5YS
Tel: 01733 758341
E-mail: shiatsu@graphic-scan.co.uk

Members have the initials: MRSS.

Relevant bodies in other English-speaking countries are:

Australian Acupuncture & Chinese Medical Association (AACMA)
PO Box 5142
West End
Brisbane
Queensland
Australia 4101

Tel: +07 3846 5866
Fax: +07 3846 5276
Free Call: 1800 025 334
E-mail: aaca@eis.net.au
Website: http://www2.eis.net.au/-aaca

**The International Institute of Chinese Medicine
and Acupuncture**
PO Box 2246
19 Av Disandt-Fresnaye
Cape Town 8000
South Africa
Tel: 27 21 434 1654

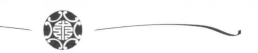

LEARNING MORE ABOUT CHINESE MEDICINE

Acupuncture and Chinese medicine in general

The Web That Has No Weaver: Understanding Chinese Medicine, Ted Kaptchuk, Congdon and Weed, New York, 1983
This is the best overall introduction to Chinese medicine for the serious layperson. It has been a standard since it was first published over a dozen years ago and it has yet to be replaced.

Clinical Handbook of Chinese Prepared Medicine, Chun-han Zhu, Paradigm Publications, Brookline, Massachusetts, 1989
This book is an excellent reference text for Chinese prepared or patent medicines. It uses a professionally accurate, standard translation, so the terminology is similar to that used in this book. It is beautifully designed and laid out and is easy to use. This is most definitely my first choice of books on Chinese patent medicines.

Chinese Medicine: Acupuncture, Herbal Remedies, Nutrition, Qui Gong and Meditation, Tom Williams, Element Health Essentials
This is a good basic introduction to the whole field of Chinese medicine for the layperson.

Acupuncture, Peter Mole, Element Books
A simple and clear introduction to acupuncture for the layperson.

A Guide to Acupuncture, Peter Firebrace and Sandra Hill, Constable Books
A comprehensive introduction to acupuncture for the layperson with some illustrations and photographs.

Between Heaven and Earth: A Guide to Chinese Medicine, Harriet Beinfield and Efrem Corngold, Ballantine Books, New York
This book is particularly good with regard to the more psychological and emotional aspects of Chinese medicine and has a good introduction to herbal medicine for the layperson.

Acupuncture in Practice, Hugh McPherson and Ted Kaptchuk (eds), Churchill Livingstone
This is a book of case histories from the West; it illustrates the wide variety of styles and methods of practice of acupuncture by many well known practitioners.

Chinese Herbal Medicine, a Practical Guide to the Healing Powers of Herbs, Dr Guang Xu, Vermillion
A good introduction to Chinese herbal medicine.

Japanese Acupuncture, a Clinical Guide, Stephen Birch and Junko Ida, Paradigm Publications
This book gives very good, clear details on moxibustion but is aimed at practitioner level.

Chinese dietary therapy
Healing with Wholefoods, Oriental Traditions and Modern Nutrition, Paul Pritchard, North Atlantic Books
A comprehensive source book for both the layperson and the professional.

Helping Ourselves: A Guide to the Traditional Chinese Food Energetics, Daverick Legget, Meridian Press
This book is designed for ease of use with its clear layout and wallcharts.

Chinese Medical Wines and Elixirs, Bob Flaws, Blue Poppy Press, Boulder, Colorado.

The Book of Jook: Chinese Medical Porridges: A Healthy Alternative to the Typical Western Breakfast, Bob Flaws, Blue Poppy Press, Boulder, Colorado.

Chinese Medicinal Teas: Simple, Proven, Folk Formulas for Common Diseases and Promoting Health, Zong Xiao-fan and Gary Liscum, Blue Poppy Press, Boulder, Colorado.

Asian psychology and psychotherapy

The Quiet Therapies: Japanese Pathways to Personal Growth, David K. Reynolds, University of Hawaii Press, Honolulu, 1987
This book is a good introduction to Japanese forms of psychotherapy based on a practical, rather than analytical approach. It also discusses the psychotherapeutic benefits of deep relaxation.
Also by the same author:
Playing Ball on Running Water
Even in Winter the Ice Doesn't Melt

Tibetan Buddhist Medicine and Psychiatry: The Diamond Healing, Terry Clifford, Samuel Weiser Inc., York Beach, ME, 1984
This book explains the Tibetan Buddhist approach to the diagnosis and treatment of mental–emotional disorders. Although Tibetan medicine is not exactly the same as Chinese medicine, they are historically related and many of the insights of Tibetan medicine in terms of psychological disorders are very profound and effective.

SUPPLIERS OF CHINESE HERBAL MEDICINES AND SPECIALIST PRODUCTS

In the UK, it is not possible to buy Chinese herbal medicines over the counter: you will need a prescription from a qualified Chinese herbalist. Some acupuncturists are able to prescribe traditional remedies or 'patents'. The suppliers listed here are members of CMAS – The Chinese Medicine Association of Suppliers. CMAS is a professional organisation which acts as a self-regulatory body to lobby in the interests of its members within the bounds of public safety. All members are subject to a code of practice. CMAS is a rapidly growing organisation so it may have more members since this list was completed.

Many of the members of CMAS have an excellent supply of books and other products relating to Chinese medicine or acupuncture. Most, if not all, suppliers have a mail-order service.

This list is by no means exhaustive. There are many other suppliers of acupuncture products and many shops that sell Chinese herbs. The acupuncture product suppliers are a good source should you wish to buy the seven-star hammer or the Japanese pure moxa mentioned in the chapter on home remedies. Please note that the Chinese herbal medicine shops one sees on many high streets may not be regulated.

Acumedic (range of products and books)
101–5 Camden High Street
London
NW1 7JN
Tel: 0171 388 5783
Fax: 0171 387 5766

Beijing Tong Ren Tang (herbal products)
124 Shaftesbury Avenue
London
W1V 7DJ
Tel: 0171 287 0098
Fax: 0171 287 0068

China Medica (herbal products)
25 Lonsdale Close
London
SE9 4HF
Tel: 0181 857 9777
Fax: 0181 480 2020

Chinese Medical Centre (herbal products)
179 South Street
Romford
Essex
RM1 1PS
Tel: 01708 756363
Fax: 01708 703015

East West Herbs (range of products and books)
Langston Priory Mews
Kingham
Oxfordshire
OX7 6UP
Tel: 01608 658862
Fax: 01608 658816
E-mail: robert@eastwestherbs.co.uk

Great Wall (herbal products)
Unit 27
Riverside Works
Hertford Road
Barking
Essex
IG11 8BN
Tel: 0181 591 6896
Fax: 0181 591 6891

Harmony Medical Distribution (range of products)
629 High Road
Leytonstone
London
E11 4PA
Tel: 0181 518 7337
Fax: 0181 556 5038
E-mail: harmony@tcm.org.uk

Lotus (herbal products)
Priorsfield Priory
Forest Row
Sussex
RH18 5HR
Tel: 01342 823053
Fax: 01342 826027
E-mail: user@lotus.u-net.com

Mayway UK (herbal products)
43 Waterside Trading Centre
Trumpers Way
Hanwell
Middlesex
Tel: 0181 893 6873
Fax: 0181 893 6874

Naturally Chinese (range of products)
P.O. Box 4584
Kiln Farm
Milton Keynes
Bucks
MK13 9BT
Tel: 0151 571 0407

Number One Herb Co. (herbal products)
36 Bankhurst Road
Catford
London
SE6 4XN
Tel: 0181 690 4840
Fax: 0181 690 4840
E-mail: jarrah@vossnet.co.uk

Oxford Medical Supplies (range of products)
Units 11 & 12
Horcott Industrial Estate
Fairford
Gloucestershire
GL7 4LX
Tel: 0800 975 8000
Fax: 0800 975 8111
E-mail: oxfordms@demon.co.uk

Shizhen TCM UK Ltd (herbal products)
50 Sandy Lane
Chorlton
Manchester
M21
Tel: 0161 881 0088
Fax: 0161 881 0888

Tian Tiao Ltd (herbal products)
85 Sullivan Way
Elstree
Herts
WD6 3DG
Tel: 0181 953 2320
Fax: 0181 953 3338

CHINESE MEDICAL GLOSSARY

Chinese medicine is a system unto itself. Its technical terms are uniquely its own and cannot be reduced to the definitions of Western medicine without destroying the very fabric and logic of Chinese medicine. Ultimately, because Chinese medicine was created in the Chinese language, Chinese medicine is really only understood in that language. Nevertheless, as Westerners try to understand Chinese medicine, we must translate the technical terms of Chinese medicine in English words. If some of these technical translations sound peculiar at first and their meaning is not immediately clear, this is because no equivalent concepts exist in everyday English.

In the past, some Western authors have erroneously translated technical Chinese medical terms using Western medical or at least quasi-scientific words in an attempt to make this system more acceptable to Western audiences. For instance, the words 'tonify' and 'sedate' are commonly seen in the Western Chinese medical literature even though, in the case of 'sedate', its meaning is completely opposite to the Chinese understanding of the word *xie*. *Xie* means to drain off something that has pooled and accumulated. That accumulation is seen as something excess, which should not be lingering where it is. Because it is accumulating somewhere where it shouldn't, it is impeding and obstructing whatever should be moving to and through that area. The word 'sedate' comes from the Latin word *sedere*, to sit. Therefore, sedate means to make something sit still. However, the Chinese *xie* means draining off that which is sitting somewhere erroneously. Therefore, to think that one is going to sedate what is already sitting is a great mistake in understanding the clinical implication and application of this technical term.

Hence, in order to preserve the integrity of this system while still making it intelligible to English-language readers, we have appended the following glossary of Chinese medical technical terms. The terms themselves are based on Nigel Wiseman's *English–Chinese Chinese–English Dictionary of Chinese Medicine* (see page 169). Dr Wiseman is, I believe, the greatest Western scholar in terms of the translation of Chinese medicine into English. Although Wiseman's terms may be awkward-sounding at first, they convey most accurately the Chinese understanding and logic of these terms.

Acquired essence: Essence manufactured out of the surplus of qi and blood in turn created out of the refined essence of food and drink

Acupoints: Those places on the channels and network vessels where qi and blood tend to collect in denser concentrations and thus those places where the qi and blood in the channels are especially available for manipulation

Acupuncture: The regulation of qi flow by the stimulation of certain points located on the channels and network vessels achieved mainly by insertion of fine needles into these points

Astringent: Constricting and containing, keeping in rather than letting go

Blood: The red-coloured fluids that flow in the vessels and nourish and construct the tissues of the body

Blood stasis: Also called dead blood, malign blood and dry blood, blood stasis is blood that is no longer moving through the vessels as it should. Instead it is precipitated in the vessels like silt in a river. It obstructs the free flow of the blood in the vessels and also impedes the production of new or fresh blood.

Blood vacuity: Insufficient blood manifesting in diminished nourishment, construction and moistening of body tissues

Bowels: The hollow yang organs of Chinese medicine

Bowstring: One of the 28 pulse qualities recognised in Chinese medicine

Burner: *see* **Triple burner**

Channels: The main routes for the distribution of qi and blood, but mainly qi

Chest oppression: A feeling of tightness and stuffiness in the chest. As a reaction to this feeling, the person will often sigh in an attempt to inhale fresh air and exhale the pent-up stale air

Choppy: One of the 28 pulse qualities recognised in Chinese medicine

Clear: The pure or clear part of ingested food and drink that is then turned into qi and blood

Cold: A pathogenic factor that can invade the body from the external environment. May combine with wind. Can also be produced as a weakness of internal physiological processes

Constructive qi: The qi that flows through the channels and nourishes and constructs the internal organs and body tissues

Counterflow: An erroneous flow of qi, usually upwards but sometimes horizontally as well

Coursing the liver: Encouraging the correct functioning of the liver viscera with regard to the flow of qi throughout the body

Damp heat: A combination of accumulated dampness mixed with pathological heat often associated with sores, abnormal vaginal discharges and some types of menstrual and body pain

Dampness: A pathological accumulation of body fluids

Decoction: A method of administering Chinese medicinals by boiling these medicinals in water, straining off the dregs and drinking the resulting medicinal liquid

Deep: One of the 28 pulse qualities recognised in Chinese medicine

Defensive qi: The yang qi that protects the exterior of the body from invasion by the environmental excesses

Depression: Stagnation and lack of movement, as in liver depression qi stagnation

Depressive heat: Pathological heat due to enduring or severe qi stagnation, which then transforms into heat

Drain: To drain off or away some pathological qi or substance from where it is replete or excess

Essence: A stored, very potent form of substance and qi, usually yin when compared to yang qi, but can be transformed into yang qi

External causes of disease: The six environmental excesses

Fine: One of the 28 pulse qualities in Chinese medicine

Fire (life gate fire, fire effulgence): A pathogenic factor that is usually created within the body

Five phase theory: An ancient Chinese system of correspondences dividing up all of reality into five phases, which then mutually engender and check each other according to definite sequences

Heat: A pathogenic factor that is usually created within the body

Heat toxins: A particularly virulent and concentrated type of pathological heat often associated with purulence (i.e. pus formation), sores and sometimes, but not always, malignancies

Hydrotherapy: Using various baths and water applications to treat and prevent disease

Impediment: A hindrance to the free flow of the qi and blood typically manifesting as pain and restriction in the range of movement of a joint or extremity

Internal causes of disease: The seven effects or emotions, namely anger, joy (or excitement), sorrow, thought, fear, melancholy and fright

Life gate fire: Another name for kidney yang or kidney fire, seen as the ultimate source of yang qi in the body

Magnet therapy: Applying magnets to acupuncture points to treat and prevent disease

Mansion: Realm of influence of one of the viscera

Moxibustion: Burning the herb Artemisia Argyium (Oriental mugwort) on, over or near acupuncture points in order to add yang qi, to warm cold, or promote the movement of the qi and blood

Network vessels: Small vessels that form a net-like web insuring the flow of qi and blood to all body tissues

Pattern discrimination: Basis for diagnosis in TCM. A pattern is determined by the signs and symptoms and observations of the individual patient's condition

Phlegm: A pathological accumulation of phlegm or mucus congealed from dampness or body fluids

Portals: Also called orifices, the openings of the sensory organs and the opening of the heart through which the spirit makes contact with the world outside

Qi: Activity, energy function, that which moves, transforms, defends, restrains and warms

Qi mechanism: The process of transforming yin substance controlled and promoted by the qi, largely synonymous with the process of digestion

Qi vacuity: An insufficiency of qi manifesting in diminished movement, transformation and function

Repletion: Excess or fullness, almost always pathological

Resolve the exterior: Release and clear the pathogens from the outer layers of the body where its primary defence mechanisms are located

Seven star hammer: A small hammer with needles embedded in its head used to stimulate acupoints without actually inserting needles

Slippery: A pulse quality, one of 28 recognised in TCM

Soggy: A pulse quality, one of 28 recognised in TCM

Spirit: The accumulation of qi in the heart that manifests as consciousness, sensory awareness and mental–emotional function

Stagnation: Non-movement of the qi, lack of free flow, constraint

Supplement: To add to or augment, as in supplementing the qi, blood, yin, or yang

Triple burner: The three areas of the abdomen, known respectively as the lower, middle and upper burners, that act as a kind of crucible within which the vital energies of the body are transformed and created by heat

Turbid: The yin, impure, turbid part of food and drink that is sent downwards to be excreted as waste

Vacuity: Emptiness or insufficiency, typically of qi, blood, yin, or yang

Vacuity cold: Obvious signs and symptoms of cold due to a lack or insufficiency of yang qi

Vacuity heat: Heat due to hyperactive yang in turn due to insufficient controlling yin

Vessels: The main routes for the distribution of qi and blood, but mainly blood

Viscera: The solid yin organs of Chinese medicine

Wind cold invasion: When the external pathogens of wind and cold have broken through the body's defences

Wind evils: External pathogenic factors, unseen pathogens that invade the body's defences

Yang: In the body, function, movement, activity and transformation

Yang vacuity: Insufficient warming and transforming function giving rise to symptoms of cold in the body

Yin: In the body, substance and nourishment

Yin vacuity: Insufficient yin substance necessary to nourish, control and counterbalance yang activity

BIBLIOGRAPHY

CHINESE LANGUAGE SOURCES

Cheng Dan An Zhen Jiu Xuan Ji (Cheng Dan An's Selected Acupuncture and Moxibustion Works), Cheng Wei-fen *et al.* (eds), Shanghai Science and Technology Press, Shanghai, 1986

Chu Zhen Zhi Liao Xue (A Study of Acupuncture Treatment), Li Zhong-yu, Sichuan Science and Technology Press, Chengdu, 1990

Fu Ke Lin Chuan Jing Hua (The Clinical Efflorescence of Gynaecology), Wang Bu-ru and Wang Qi-ming, Sichuan Science and Technology Press, Chengdu, 1989

Fu Ke Yu Chi (The Jade Ruler of Gynaecology), Shen Jin-ao, Shanghai Science and Technology Press, Shanghai, 1983

Fu Ke Zheng Zhi (Gynaecological Patterns and Treatments), Sun Jiu-ling, Hebei People's Press, 1983

Gu Fang Miao Yong (Ancient Formulas, Wondrous Uses), Chen Bao-ming and Zhao Jin-xi, Science and Technology Popularization Press, Beijing, 1994

Han Ying Chang Yong Yi Xue Ci Hui (Chinese–English Glossary of Commonly Used Medical Terms), Huang Xiao-kai, People's Health and Hygiene Press, Beijing, 1982

Nan Zhi Bing De Liang Fang Miao Fa (Fine Formulas and Wondrous Methods for Difficult to Treat Diseases), Wu Da-zhen and He Xin-qiao, Chinese National Medicine and Medicinal Press, Beijing, 1992

Nei Ke Bing Liang Fang (Internal Medicine Disease Fine Formulas), He Yuan-lin and Jiang Chang-yuan, Yunnan University Press, Zhongqing, 1991

Qi Nan Za Zheng Jing (Carefully Chosen Curious, Difficult, Miscellaneous Diseases), Huang Bing-yuan, Guangdong Science and Technology Press, Guangzhou, 1996

Shang Hai Lao Zhong Yi Jing Yan Xuan Bian (A Selected Compilation of Shanghai Old Doctors' Experiences), Shanghai Science and Technology Press, Shanghai, 1984

Shi Yong Zhen Jiu Tui Na Zhi Liao Xue (A Study of Practical Acupuncture, Moxibustion and Tui Na Treatments), Xia Zhi-ping, Shanghai College of Chinese Medicine Press, Shanghai, 1990

Tan Zheng Lun (Treatise on Phlegm Conditions), Hou Tian-yin and Wang Chun-hua, People's Army Press, Beijing, 1989

Xian Dai Nan Zhi Bing Zhong Yi Zhen Liao Xue (A Study of the Chinese Medical Diagnosis and Treatment of Modern Difficult to Treat Diseases), Wu Jun-yu and Bai Yong-bo, Chinese Medicine Ancient Books Press, Beijing, 1993

Xue Guan Shen Jing Xing Tou Tong De Zhong Yi Zhi Liao (The Chinese Medical Treatment of Neurovascular Headaches), Feng Cun-wei, *XIn Zhong Yi (New Chinese Medicine)*, No. 9, 1996

Yi Zong Jin Jian (The Golden Mirror of Ancestral Medicine), Wu Qian *et al.*, People's Health and Hygiene Press, Beijing, 1985

Yu Xue Zheng Zhi (Static Blood Patterns and Treatments), Zhang Xue-wen, Shanxi Science and Technology Press, Xian, 1986

Zhen Jiu Chu Fang Xue (A Study of Acupuncture and Moxibustion Prescriptions), Wang Dai, Beijing Publishing Co., Beijing, 1990

Zhen Jiu Da Cheng (A Great Compendium of Acupuncture and Moxibustion), Yang Ji-zhou, People's Health and Hygiene Press, Beijing, 1983

Zhen Jiu Xue (A Study of Acupuncture and Moxibustion), Qiu Mao-liang *et al.*, Shanghai Science and Technology Press, Shanghai, 1985

Zhen Jiu Yi Xue (An Easy Study of Acupuncture and Moxibustion), Li Shou-xian, People's Health and Hygiene Press, Beijing, 1990

Zhong Guo Min Jian Cao Yao Fang (Chinese Folk Herbal

Medicinal Formulas), Liu Guang-rui and Liu Shao-lin, Sichuan Science and Technology Press, Chengdu, 1992

Zhong Guo Zhen Jiu Chu Fang Xue (A Study of Chinese Acupuncture and Moxibustion Prescriptions), Xiao Shao-qing, Ningxia People's Press, Yinchuan, 1986

Zhong Guo Zhong Yi Mi Fang Da Quan (A Great Compendium of Chinese National Chinese Medical Secret Formulas), Hu Zhao-ming (ed.), Literary Propagation Publishing Company, Shanghai, 1992

Zhong Yi Bing Yin Bing Ji Xue (A Study of Chinese Medical Disease Causes and Disease Mechanisms), Wu Dun-xu, Shanghai College of Chinese Medicine Press, Shanghai, 1989

Zhong Yi Fu Ke Zhi Liao Shou Ce (A Handbook of Chinese Medical Gynaecological Treatment), Wu Shi-xing and Qi Cheng-lin, Shanxi Science and Technology Press, Xian, 1991

Zhong Yi Hu Li Xue (A Study of Chinese Medical Nursing), Lu Su-ying, People's Health and Hygiene Press, Beijing, 1983

Zhong Yi Lin Chuang Ge Ke (Various Clinical Specialties in Chinese Medicine), Zhang En-qin *et al.*, Shanghai College of Chinese Medicine Press, Shanghai, 1990

Zhong Yi Ling Yan Fang (Efficacious Chinese Medical Formulas), Lin Bin-zhi, Science and Technology Propagation Press, Beijing, 1991

Zhong Yi Miao Yong Yu Yang Sheng (Chinese Medicine Wondrous Uses and Nourishing Life), Ni Qi-lan, Liberation Army Press, Beijing, 1993

Zhong Yi Nei Ke Lin Chuang Shou Ce (A Clinical Manual of Chinese Medicine Internal Medicine), Xia De-shu, Shanghai Science and Technology Press, Shanghai, 1990

Zhong Yi Nei Ke Xue (The Study of Chinese Medicine Internal Medicine), Zhang Bo-ying *et al.*, Shanghai Science and Technology Press, Shanghai, 1990

ENGLISH LANGUAGE SOURCES

A Barefoot Doctor's Manual, revised and enlarged edition, Cloudburst Press, Mayne Isle, 1977

'Acupuncture in the Treatment of Migraine', G. Kukiena, *Fortschritte Der Medezin,* Vol. 103, No. 25, July 4, 1985

'Acupuncture in the Treatment of Migraine', Y.K. Batra, *American Journal of Acupuncture,* Vol. 14, No. 2, June 1986

'Acupuncture for Long-term Treatment of Headache in a National Health Center', Y.K. Sapo Junnila, *American Journal of Acupuncture,* Vol 14, No. 4, Dec. 1986

'Acupuncture in the Prophylactic Treatment of Migraine Headache: A Pilot Study', L. Lenhard and P.M.E. Waite, *New Zealand Medical Journal,* Vol. 96, No. 738, 1983

'Acupuncture versus Medical Treatment for Migraine and Muscle Tension Headache', L. Loh, P.W. Nathan, G.D. Schott, K.J. Zilkha, *Journal of Neurology, Neurosurgery, and Psychiatry,* Vol. 47, No. 4, 1984.

Chinese–English Terminology of Traditional Chinese Medicine, Shuai Xue-zhong *et al.,* Hunan Science and Technology Press, Changsha, 1983

Chinese–English Manual of Commonly-used Prescriptions in Traditional Chinese Medicine, Ou Ming (ed.), Joint Publishing Co. Ltd, Hong Kong, 1989

Chinese Herbal Medicine: Formulas and Strategies, Dan Bensky and Randall Barolet, Eastland Press, Seattle, 1990

Chinese Herbal Medicine: Materia Medica, Dan Bensky and Andrew Gamble, second (revised) edition, Eastland Press, Seattle, 1993

Chinese Self-massage, The Easy Way to Health, Fan Ya-li, Blue Poppy Press, Boulder, Colorado, 1996

A Clinical Guide to Chinese Herbs and Formulae, Cheng Song-yu and Li Fei, Churchill and Livingstone, Edinburgh, 1993

A Clinical Manual of Chinese Herbal Medicine and Acupuncture, Zhou Zhong Ying and Jin Hui De, Churchill Livingstone, Edinburgh, 1997

A Compendium of TCM Patterns and Treatments, Bob Flaws and Daniel Finney, Blue Poppy Press, Boulder, Colorado, 1996

A Comprehensive Guide to Chinese Herbal Medicine, Chen Ze-lin and Chen Mei-fang, Oriental Healing Arts Institute, Long Beach, California, 1992

English–Chinese Chinese–English Dictionary of Chinese Medicine, Nigel Wiseman, Hunan Science and Technology Press, Changsha, 1995

Fundamentals of Chinese Acupuncture, Andrew Ellis, Nigel Wiseman and Ken Boss, Paradigm Publications, Brookline, Massachusetts, 1988

Fundamentals of Chinese Medicine, Nigel Wiseman and Andrew Ellis, Paradigm Publications, Brookline, Massachusetts, 1985

Glossary of Chinese Medical Terms and Acupuncture Points, Nigel Wiseman and Ken Boss, Paradigm Publications, Brookline, Massachusetts, 1990

Handbook of Chinese Herbs and Formulas, Him-che Yeung, self-published, Los Angeles, 1985

A Handbook of Differential Diagnosis with Key Signs and Symptoms, Therapeutic Principles and Guiding Prescriptions, Ou-yang Yi, (trans. C.S. Cheung), Harmonious Sunshine Cultural Centre, San Francisco, 1987

How to Find Relief from Migraine, Rosemary Dudley and Wade Rowland, Beaufort Books Inc., New York City/Toronto, 1982

Mastering Your Migraine, Peter Evans, E.P. Dutton, New York, 1979

Migraines and Headaches, Understanding, Controlling, and Avoiding the Pain, Marcia Wilkinson, Arco Publishing, New York, 1982

Migraine and Other Headaches, James W. Lance, Charles Scribner's Sons, New York, 1986

Migraine, The Breakthrough Study that Explains What Causes It and How It Can Be Completely Prevented Through Diet, Rodolfo Low, Henry Holt and Co., New York, 1987

Migraine, The Evolution of a Common Disorder, Oliver W. Sacks, University of California Press, Berkeley, 1970

Migraine, The Facts, F. Clifford Rose and M. Gavel, Oxford University Press, New York, 1979

Migraine, Understanding a Common Disorder, Oliver W. Sacks, University of California Press, Berkeley, 1985

Oriental Materia Medica, A Concise Guide, Hong-yen Hsu, Oriental Healing Arts Institute, Long Beach, California, 1986

Practical Therapeutics of Traditional Chinese Medicine, Yan Wu and Warren Fischer, Paradigm Publications, Brookline, Massachusetts, 1997

Practical Traditional Chinese Medicine and Pharmacology: Clinical Experiences, Shang Xian-min *et al.,* New World Press, Beijing, 1990

Practical Traditional Chinese Medicine and Pharmacology: Herbal Formulas, Geng Jun-ying, *et al.,* New World Press, Beijing, 1991

The English–Chinese Encyclopaedia of Practical Traditional Chinese Medicine, Vol. 12: Gynaecology, Xuan Jia-sheng (ed.), Higher Education Press, Beijing, 1990

The Essential Book of Traditional Chinese Medicine, Vol. 2: Clinical Practice, Liu Yan-chi, (trans. Fang Ting-yu and Chen Lai-di), Columbia University Press, New York, 1988

The Foundations of Chinese Medicine, Giovanni Maciocia, Churchill Livingstone, Edinburgh, 1989

The Merck Manual, 15th edition, Robert Berkow (ed.), Merck Sharp and Dohme Research Laboratories, Rahway, New Jersey, 1987

The Practice of Chinese Medicine, Giovanni Maciocia, Churchill Livingstone, Edinburgh, 1994

The Treatment of Disease in TCM, Volume 1: Diseases of the Head and Face Including Mental/Emotional Disorders, Philippe Sionneau and Lu Gang, Blue Poppy Press, Boulder, Colorado, 1996

Traditional Medicine in Contemporary China, Nathan Sivin, University of Michigan, Ann Arbor, 1987

Zang Fu: The Organ Systems of Traditional Chinese Medicine (second edition), Jeremy Ross, Churchill Livingstone, Edinburgh, 1985.

INDEX

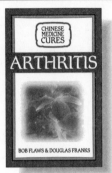

October 1999 -
Chinese Medicine Cures Arthritis -
ISBN: 0-572-02540-8

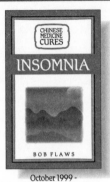

October 1999 -
Chinese Medicine Cures Insomnia -
ISBN: 0-572-02568-8

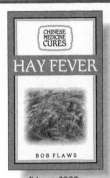

February 2000 -
Chinese Medicine Cures Hayfever -
ISBN: 0-572-02576-9

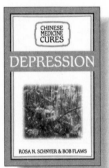

February 2000 -
Chinese Medicine Cures Depression -
ISBN: 0-572-02577-7

CHINESE MEDICINE CURES

BY WORLD-RENOWNED EXPERT
BOB FLAWS
Governor of the National Academy of
Acupuncture and Oriental Medicine
Fellow of The Register of
Chinese Herbal Medicine.
Edited by
Sylvia Schroer BSc MRCHM MBAcC
Council Member of the
Register of Chinese Medicine

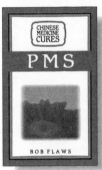

Summer 2000 -
Chinese Medicine Cures PMS - ISBN:
0-572-02539-4

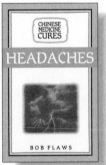

Summer 2000 -
Chinese Medicine Cures Headaches -
ISBN: 0-572-02590-4

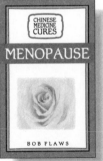

Autumn 2000 -
Chinese Medicine Cures Menopause -
ISBN: 0-572-02591-2

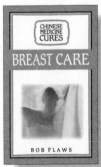

Autumn 2000 -
Chinese Medicine Cures Breast Care-
ISBN: 0-572-02592-0